A larger font is used in this book to accommodate those whose eyesight may be fading.

Natural Weight Loss and Diabetes Control
The Medical Librarian's Annotated Guide

By William Jiang, MLS

New York

This is a work of nonfiction. None of the passages in this book should be understood or construed as a recommendation or condemnation of any particular drug, medication, or treatment for mental illness.

For information, address kd3qc@yahoo.com
Designed by William Jiang
Jiang, William 1972-
Natural Weight Loss and Diabetes Control: The Medical Librarian's Annotated Guide /
William Jiang
183p.19.8cm.
ISBN-13: 978-1533620750
ISBN-10: 153362075X
1. Health-- Weight Loss

Table of Contents

Introduction

Natural Weight Loss and Diabetes Control: Food-stuffs and Nutraceuticals

Top Recommendations for Dietary Change to Achieve Successful Weight-Loss and Natural Diabetes Control

- Magnesium- It's good for what ails you
- A Mix of Helpful Nutrients- And an Insulin Mimetic
- Fiber, Weight Loss, and Diabetes Control

World Cuisines and Traditional Styles of Healthy Eating

The Hunter-Gatherer Diet- The Good Old Days
- Organic Veggies are Richer in Nutrients
- Meat Raised Without Antibiotics or Hormones
- Locally Grown Foodstuffs are Best
- Berries and Health
- Nuts about Nuts
- Coconut: The All-Giving Tree

The Mediterranean Diet
- **The Biblical and Middle Eastern Roots of the Mediterranean Diet**
- **The Mediterranean diet is great for keeping a healthy weight**
- **Olive Oil and Inflammation**
- **The Mediterranean Diet: On the Genomic Level**

The Asian Diet and Maintaining a Healthy Weight
- Green Tea and Weight Loss
- Seaweed and Weight Loss
- Turmeric, Onions, Garlic

Components of the Traditional Latin American Healthy Diet
- Beans and Health
- Avocados- good for the heart and Nervous System

- Chocolate and Heart Health

Components of the European Healthy Diet
- Red Wine, Resveratrol and Apigenin
- Polyphenols

Components of A Healthy Diet from Africa and the Middle East
- Coffee
- African Mango?
- Black Seed

The Role of Fruit, Veggies, and Fermentation in Weight Loss and Natural Diabetes Control
- The Meaning of Fruit and Vegetable Colors
- Citrus and Weight Loss
- Grapefruit and Weight Loss
- Kale, Cabbage, Collard Greens, Brussel Sprouts: the Brassica Vegetables
- Apples and Weight Loss
- Fermented Fruits and Vegetables and Health
- Yogurt and Kefir do a Body Good
- Vinegar and Weight Loss

Nutraceuticals

- CoQ10
- Vitamin D
- Vitamin E
- Zinc
- Carnitine
- Taurine
- Turmeric
- Calcium

Foods to Minimize
- Salt
- Wheat and Anti-Nutrients
- Trans Fats and Weight Gain
- Eating Fast Food Causes Weight Gain

The Role of Exercise in Weight Loss and Diabetes Management

- Strength Training and Basal Metabolism Rate (BMR)
- Brown Fat and Basal Metabolism Rate
- Reducing White Fat with Arginine
- Walking and Bicycling
- Is Sitting at Your Computer Killing You?
- The Possible Benefits of Standing Desks
- Yoga and Weight Loss
- Mindful Eating and Weight Loss
- Long Term Meditation and Yoga and Basal Metabolic Rate
- Thirty Minutes of Exercise Enough to Strengthen The Body on a Cellular Level

Other Aspects of Weight Management that are Important but Often Overlooked

- Complementary and Alternative Traditional Treatments (CAM) of High Blood Sugar
- Apps and Weight Loss
- Belief in God Protects the Faithful
- A Glass of Alcohol Daily will give you a longer, healthier life
- Living in Polluted Cities can Cause Asthma, Liver and Heart Damage

Introduction

Mens sana in corpore sano is a Latin phrase, usually translated as "a sound mind in a sound body" or "a healthy mind in a healthy body", is attributed to the Roman poet, Juvenal who lived during the first century AD. The link between body and mind has been known for over two thousand years, and yet we think we can eat that Big Mac and not suffer consequences. There is a strong link between that fast food and obesity, diabetes, clinical depression, and other serious problems of body and mind.. Indeed, even clinical depression and schizophrenia can possibly be prevented by a healthy diet. For an interesting book about natural mental health I invite you to check out my ***Guide to Natural Mental Health: Anxiety, Bipolar, Depression, Schizophrenia, and Digital Addiction: Nutrition, and Complementary Therapies, 3rd Edition***.

A word of caution: one should **ALWAYS** check an individual vitamin or supplement against your medical condition list, such as diabetes or high blood pressure, and also each nutraceutical should be checked against the medications and other vitamins and minerals one is taking. For example, if somebody has high blood pressure, it would behoove them to avoid salt, or alternatively there may be an interaction between their heart medicine and grapefruit juice. Also, it is a good rule to change one nutraceutical or strategy at a time, rather than changing around everything, all at once. That way, you know what works for you and what does not. Also, one should always take the USDA Recommended Daily Allowance (RDA) or minimum effective dose of any of the natural interventions I list in this book. Why?

Even too much water can be lethal. If you megadose on neurosteroids, vitamins, minerals, or amino acids, or mix them in a dangerous way, you can do a lot of damage to yourself. That being said, I include the obligatory disclaimer here.

Disclaimer: This information is not intended to be used as a replacement for a medical doctor's advice. All information has been acquired from reputable sources, and I will personally assume no liability from any use or misuse of this information.

This book is what librarians call an annotated bibliography. This annotated bibliography picks the "best" information from the medical literature, sometimes includes commentary as well as the source, title, authors, and abstract of the article from MEDLINE. In this case, the strength of this particular annotated bibliography is the concentration of the knowledge of more than six hundred world-class experts from many medical disciplines and more than approximately two thousand support staff, all in one small volume, with **FREE FULLTEXT** often available for more in-depth reading and learning. In other words, do not take my word for anything, take the word of the almost three thousand medical researchers and allied health workers whose amazing work I've included in this small manual.

Healthy eating starts at home. In the United States, in the first quarter of 2016, almost 158 billion dollars was spent in eateries, outside of home, such as McDonalds or more upscale places. About 152 billion dollars was spent on groceries during the same time period of the first quarter of 2016. So, for the first time in the history of the United States, people spent more money eating out than eating at home.

Mostly this growth in numbers of people eating out has been spurred by millennials, the youngest of adults.

Concurrently, suicides are at a thirty-year high, as of April 2016. Obviously, there are many reasons for the abnormally high suicide rate beyond eating out. To truly understand why suicide is at a peak as this book is being ritten, one would have to dissect the the social, economic, technological, political, and stressful modern lives in which we live. However, the more people that eat out at McDonalds and other fast food restaurants, the unhealthier their bodies as well as their brains become. See the documentaries **Supersize Me** and **Food Inc** if you need inspiration to eat healthy.

Varying the diet in a healthy way is best. This book presents many healthy dietary options to choose from. For example, grapefruit can help people lose weight. However, that does not mean to eat only grapefruit all the time. When the diet is varied, the gut microbiome is healthier. A problem in today's world is that our diets are not as varied as our ancestors were. This can be changed.

The information found in this book about Natural Weight Loss and Diabetes Control should be talked over with your medical provider. The information presented is meant as a guide for discovery. The good news is that there is much that can be done to get to and maintain a healthy weight as well as diabetes control, with the aid of your nutritionist and your medical team.

The World Wide Web

Indeed, there is a "chicken and egg" relationship between depression and ten of the top ten causes of death in the United States, where sometimes depression comes before the physical disease or vice-versa. Clinical depression is mixed with: cancer, heart disease, asthma, chronic stress, stroke, diabetes, Alzheimer's and other dementias, kidney disease, and yes even suicide. The only top causes of death that

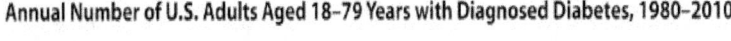

Annual Number of U.S. Adults Aged 18–79 Years with Diagnosed Diabetes, 1980–2010

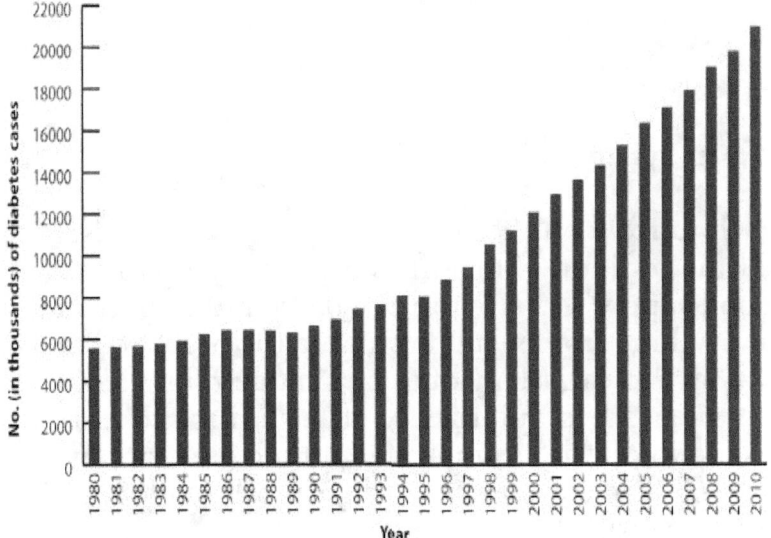

Source: National Diabetes Surveillance System, National Health Interview Survey data.

What happened in 1994 to precipitate this meteoric increase in diabetes? Did our eating habits change? Our basic biology? No. Tim Berners-Lee debuted the World Wide Web in 1994 at the European physics laboratory, CERN.

All technologies are a doubled edged sword, since

fire came on the world stage. Fire warmed our living spaces and cooked our food, and it was used to burn our houses to the ground during war or misuse. So it is with the greatest technological advance in education and communication since movable type, the World Wide Web. As a society, we sit at our desks far too long and we use our computers far too much to be healthy. Even at night we find ourselves drawn to the friendly glow of the computer screen, to Facebook or to do other things.

Corn Syrup

Before 1994 our health was not so good, because of the addition of high fructose corn syrup to the food supply. Corn Syrup can be found in practically everything from salad dressing to the processed meats we love to eat. Many of today's modern ills are due to the nearly omnipresence of high fructose corn syrup in our food supply. High Fructose Corn Syrup HFCS is in almost all of today's processed foodstuffs. From Wikipedia:

Obesity and metabolic disorders

Sugars became a health concern among the American public in the early 1970s with the publication of John Yudkin's book, Pure, White and Deadly, which claimed that simple sugars, an increasingly large part of the Western diet, were dangerous. In the 1980s and 1990s Gerald Reaven and Sheldon Reiser of the USDA published papers discussing the dangers of dietary fructose from consumption of sucrose and of HFCS, especially with regard to heart disease, diabetes, and obesity. These concerns came to the public's attention through media attention to a 2004 commentary in The American Journal of Clinical Nutrition that suggested that the altered metabolism of fructose when compared to glucose may be a factor in increasing obesity rates since, as compared to glucose, fructose may be more readily converted to fat and the sugar causes less of a rise in insulin and leptin, both of which increase feelings of satiety. Fructose, in contrast to glucose, was shown to potently stimulate lipogenesis (creation of fatty acids, for conversion to fat).

Bleached White Flour

What else can we add to this ridiculous mountain of maladies? Even before the introduction of corn syrup in the 1970s, bleached white flour was on the scene beginning in 1875. In the late 19th and early 20th centuries bleached white flour produced horrible effects on public health- including madness, caused by a yet unknown vitamin deficiency in the diet. This new disease was called pellagra.

Why did the disease of pellagra arise at that point in time? Created partly due to economic forces, a new

17

milling technology called a steel "roller flour mill" made it possible to make cheap, non-nutritive white flour in bulk. The new roller flour mill technology became widespread in part due to European demand for cheap American flour. The roller flour mill technology takes the bran and other healthful parts of the wheat and extracts it, leaving behind delicious yet unhealthy, white flour. It tasted good, it was inexpensive, sure but it caused many to be locked up in asylums, until death, Ironically, pellagra is a disease which is easily treated by a nutritious diet. Read on for the history of and scientifically discovered cause and subsequent cure of pellagra, straight from the historical archives of the New York Times, the "Paper of Record".

Published: September 8, 1916
FIND PELLAGRA CURE IN CHANGE OF DIET: Federal Health Service Experiments in Orphan Asylums Remove Odium from Some Foods FLOUR MAKERS SUFFERED Consumption of Highly Milled Product Fell Off 25 Per Cent. Under Misconception of the Facts.
Special to The New York Times.

WASHINGTON, Sept. 7.—An experiment just concluded by the Public Health Service at two orphan asylums at Jackson, Miss., has demonstrated that the disease known as pellagra, the appearance of which in this country caused some alarm and considerable discussion, can be cured by proper dietary measures and has shown apparently that it is not due to any one article of food, but to an "unbalanced" diet. The Public Health Service released the subjects at the two asylums for Governmental observation on Sept. 1, approximately two years after the beginning of the experiment.

The outcome of the experiment is important in view of a statement by the publishers of the American Miller that, as a result of an official publication on the subject of pellagra, last April, the production of highly milled flours had fallen off nearly 25 per cent., and the flour industry had been hit hard in a financial way. At the Public Health Service headquarters the explanation is made that an article in one of the reports of the service was misinterpreted to mean that the use of highly milled flour had been discovered as the cause of pellagra. An entirely erroneous construction was placed on this article, it was said, and in order to correct the misconception the Public Health Service has made a statement reading as follows:

"In the Public Health reports for April 14, 1916, there appeared an article under the following heading: 'Bread as a Food,' with a sub-heading: 'Changes in Its Vitamin Content and Nutritive Value with Reference to the Occurrence of Pellagra.'

"The facts set forth as regards pellagra have not been challenged, but as some erroneous inferences concerning the value of white flour and of bread made from it have been drawn from the paper, it appears desirable to submit the following statement:

"The paper referred to presented the results of certain of the studies which are being made on pellagra and was designed to demonstrate primarily that when a diet poor in essential food elements, aside from cereals, was constantly used it appeared likely that if the carbohydrate element contained a liberal amount of the accessory food substance known to be contained in whole grains the probability of pellagra developing was less than when the starchy element of food was deficient in these substances.

A Mixed Diet Necessary.

"From the broad view of nutrition, it is very probably immaterial what kind of flour is used in making bread provided that an adequate mixed diet is consumed which will supply sufficient of the essential dietary components outside of the cereals contained in the diet. It may be added that the great majority of people in this country live on a well-balanced, sufficient, mixed diet."

In the early stages of the investigation of pellagra in this country the theory was advanced that the disease was due to the use of corn meal. In the recent experiments of the Public Health Service cornmeal has been employed in the curative diet prescribed, and cures have been effected, thus bearing out the conclusion that pellagra is not due to any one article of diet, but to the failure to use a well-balanced diet—that is, a diversified diet.

Perhaps a better illustration of what this means can be obtained from a statement in the article, "Bread as a Food," that pellagra made its appearance in southwestern France in 1820, a period followed by extreme poverty, when the people lived on cereals, fat pork, and a few fresh vegetables, but began to disappear with improved economic conditions in 1860, simultaneously with an improvement in the diet of the people, which now includes more meat, milk, and eggs. At the present time pellagra is practically unknown in France.

In a bulletin on the subject of its observation of the inmates of the two orphan asylums in Jackson, Miss., Surgeon Joseph Goldberger and Assistant Surgeon C. H. Waring of the Public Health Service say:

"The conclusion is drawn that pellagra may be prevented by an appropriate diet without any alteration in the environment, hygienic or sanitary."

The impression, which the Public Health Service says is erroneous, that it made the statement that pellagra was caused by the use of highly milled flour is supposed to have been drawn from an explanation of experiments on fowls made by officers of the service. Fowls, it was said, would live for many months in perfect health on an exclusive diet of wheat, corn, whole-wheat flour, or so-called water-ground corn meal, but if they were fed on highly milled products they would die within a month or two of polyneuritis, a disease very similar to beri beri.

The experiments have shown, however, that chickens can be cured of this disease by giving them a better-balanced diet.

The experiments conducted on the inmates of the two asylums at Jackson were begun two years ago, and the Public Health Service investigators were satisfied after a year of observation that they had demonstrated that the disease, which had existed in the institutions for some time, could be cured by employing a well-balanced diet. But, to make assurance doubly sure, the investigators continued their observation for another year, and have now released their patients from observation with the knowledge that cures are readily effected by proper diet.

Disease Long a Puzzle.

Pellagra has been one of the most puzzling diseases ever studied by medical investigators. For 200 years it has ravaged southern Europe, particularly Italy, where it has been so prevalent that it has often been called "Italian leprosy." The disease in this country has been known for about sixty years; but only in the last decade, when it has attacked thousands of people in the South, has it become a serious problem.

First manifesting itself in lassitude and intestinal disorders, pellagra affects the skin so that it finally becomes thickened and pigmented. Emaciation then sets in. The tongue and mouth later are attacked, swallowing is difficult and painful, and as a result the patient is usually delirious. Likewise the mentality is affected. Melancholia comes with a general retardation of ideas, often accompanied by suicidal tendencies.

Roughly, there have been two different theories as to the cause of pellagra. One group of investigators believed that it was communicated by an insect, while others were convinced that it was of a dietary origin. Italian scientists under Professor Lombroso of Turin, asserted that pellagra was due to the consumption of moldy corn. In this country with the alarming increase of pellagra in the South, the Public Health Service established a laboratory for observation of the disease at Columbia, S. C. In 1912, the Thompson-MacFadden Pellagra Commission, organized through the donation of $15,000 by Colonel Robert M. Thompson of New York, and John H. MacFadden of Philadelphia, set up a field headquarters in Spartensburg County, S. C. Some of the members of this commission, particularly Dr. Louis Sambon, lecturer to the London School of Tropical Medicine, arrived at the conclusion that pellagra was due not to inferior grades of corn, but to some insect carrier.

After careful study of flies and mosquitos Dr. Sambon was led to believe that the buffalo gnat was this carrier. Dr. Sambon's theory receives some support in the September issue of The American Journal of Clinical Medicine in a letter written by Dr. W. J. W. Kerr, who was surgeon in charge of the Andersonville prison hospital, Andersonville, Ga., during the civil war. Dr. Kerr says there were more than 10,000 deaths from pellagra at the prison.

"We examined everything we could conceive as being the possible cause," he writes, "and finally came to the conclusion that the whole thing was produced through the insanitary and crowded condition of the prison. Three regiments of Confederates were guarding the prison, and not one of them ever had pellagra.

"I had from 300 to 500 prisoners out on parole, and not a single case ever occurred outside of the prison after the men had been out a week or ten days. No surgeon or any one on the outside ever took the disease—yet we all had exactly the same diet. We could not get anything else, so you see that if it had been cornmeal and bad provisions the men on the outside would have had the disease precisely as those on the inside of the prison."

Dr. Edward Jenner Wood of Wilmington, N. C., who has investigated several hundred pellagra cases, came to the conclusion in the May 6 (1916) issue of The Journal of the American Medical Association that pellagra was due to the improper milling of cornmeal, but Dr. George L. Servoss, editor of The Western Medical Times, who was formerly in the milling process business, pointed out that the milling process mentioned by Dr. Wood was not the one used in the corn-milling industry, but in the manufacture of brewers' grits.

The new theory is that pellagra should be placed in the same category as beriberi, scurvy, and rickets, which are believed to be caused by a lack of vitamins or the essential constituents necessary for a well-balanced diet.

***

Healthy Diet, Healthy Psychology

As may be inferred from the previous article about pellagra, a nutritious diet leads not only to a healthy body, but also a healthy mind.

Source: PLoS One. 2016 Jan 15;11(1):e0146888.
doi: 10.1371/journal.pone.0146888. eCollection
2016.

Tite: Combined Healthy Lifestyle Is Associated with Psychological Disorders among Adults.

Authors: Saneei P1,2,3, Esmaillzadeh A1,3,4, Keshteli AH5,6, Reza Roohafza H7, Afshar H7, Feizi A6,8, Adibi P6.

Abstract: BACKGROUND AND AIMS: Joint association of lifestyle-related factors and mental health has been less studied in earlier studies, especially in Middle Eastern countries. This study aimed to examine how combinations of several lifestyle-related factors related to depression and anxiety in a large group of middle-age Iranian population.
METHODS: In a cross-sectional study on 3363 Iranian adults, a healthy lifestyle score was constructed by the use of data from dietary intakes, physical activity, smoking status, psychological distress and obesity. A dish-based 106-item semi-quantitative validated food frequency questionnaire (FFQ), General Practice Physical Activity Questionnaire (GPPAQ), General Health Questionnaire (GHQ) and other pre-tested questionnaires were used to assess the components of healthy lifestyle score. The Hospital Anxiety and Depression Scale (HADS) was applied to screen for anxiety and depression.
RESULTS: After adjustment for potential confounders, we found that individuals with the highest score of healthy lifestyle were 95% less likely to be anxious (OR: 0.05; 95% CI: 0.01-0.27) and 96% less likely to be depressed (OR: 0.04; 95% CI: 0.01-0.15), compared with those with the lowest score. In addition, non-smokers had lower odds of anxiety (OR: 0.64; 95% CI: 0.47-0.88) and depression (OR: 0.62;

95% CI: 0.48-0.81) compared with smokers. Individuals with low levels of psychological distress had expectedly lower odds of anxiety (OR: 0.13; 95% CI: 0.10-0.16) and depression (OR: 0.10; 95% CI: 0.08-0.12) than those with high levels. Individuals with a healthy diet had 29% lower odds of depression (OR: 0.71; 95% CI: 0.59-0.87) than those with a non-healthy diet.

CONCLUSION: We found evidence indicating that healthy lifestyle score was associated with lower odds of anxiety and depression in this group of Iranian adults. Healthy diet, psychological distress, and smoking status were independent predictors of mental disorders.

Glycemic Index, Glycemic Load, and FDA MyPlate

Glycemic Index

From Wikipedia, the free encyclopedia

The glycemic index or glycaemic index (GI) is a number associated with a particular type of food that indicates the food's effect on a person's blood glucose (also called blood sugar) level. A value of 100 represents the standard, an equivalent amount of pure glucose. The GI represents the total rise in a person's blood sugar level following consumption of the food; it may or may not represent the rapidity of the rise in blood sugar. The steepness of the rise can be influenced by a number of other factors, such as the quantity of fat eaten with the food. The GI is useful for understanding how the body breaks down carbohydrates and only takes into account the available carbohydrate (total carbohydrate minus fiber) in a food. Although the food may contain fats and other components that contribute to the total rise in blood sugar, these effects are not reflected in the GI.

The glycemic index is usually applied in the context of the quantity of the food and the amount of carbohydrate in the food that is actually consumed. A related measure, the glycemic load (GL), factors this in by multiplying the glycemic index of the food in question by the carbohydrate content of the actual serving. Watermelon has a high glycemic index, but a low glycemic load for the quantity typically consumed. Fructose, by contrast, has a low glycemic index, but can have a high glycemic load if a large quantity is consumed.

GI tables are available that list many types of foods and their GIs. Some tables also include the serving size and the glycemic load of the food per serving.

A practical limitation of the glycemic index is that it does not measure insulin production due to rises in blood sugar. As a result, two foods could have the same glycemic index, but produce different amounts of insulin. Likewise, two foods could have the same glycemic load, but cause different insulin responses. Furthermore, both the glycemic index and glycemic load measurements are defined by the carbohydrate content of food. For example, when eating steak, which has no carbohydrate content but provides a high protein intake, up to 50% of that protein can be converted to glucose when there is little to no carbohydrate consumed with it.

Glycemic load

From Wikipedia, the free encyclopedia
The glycemic load (GL) of food is a number that estimates how much the food will raise a person's blood glucose level after eating it. One unit of glycemic load approximates the effect of consuming one gram of glucose. Glycemic load accounts for how much carbohydrate is in the food and how much each gram of carbohydrate in the food raises blood glucose levels. Glycemic load is based on the glycemic index (GI), and is calculated by multiplying the grams of available carbohydrate in the food times the food's GI and then dividing by 100.

Glycemic load estimates the impact of carbohydrate consumption using the glycemic index while taking into account the amount of carbohydrate that is consumed. GL is a GI-weighted measure of carbohydrate content. For instance, watermelon has a high GI, but a typical serving of watermelon does not contain much carbohydrate, so the glycemic load of eating it is low. Whereas glycemic index is defined for each type of food, glycemic load can be calculated for any size serving of a food, an entire meal, or an entire day's meals.

FDA MyPlate
http://www.choosemyplate.gov

MyPlate is a reminder to find your healthy eating style and build it throughout your lifetime. Everything you eat and drink matters. The right mix can help you be healthier now and in the future. This means:

- Focus on variety, amount, and nutrition.
- Choose foods and beverages with less saturated fat, sodium, and added sugars.
- Start with small changes to build healthier eating styles.
- Support healthy eating for everyone.

Eating healthy is a journey shaped by many factors, including our stage of life, situations, preferences, access to food, culture, traditions, and the personal decisions we make over time. All your food and beverage choices count. MyPlate offers ideas and tips to help you create a healthier eating style that meets your individual needs and improves your health.

Natural Weight Loss and Diabetes Control: Foodstuffs and Nutraceuticals

"Let food be thy medicine and medicine be thy food."
- Hippocrates

The following few articles focus on the history of diabetes as well as interconnections between diet, diabetes, and other aspects of health from a micro as well as macro view.

Depression, Weight Gain, Diabetes, and Heart Disease: The Connections

FREE FULLTEXT
Source: Front Psychiatry. 2016 Mar 21;7:33. doi: 10.3389/fpsyt.2016.00033. eCollection 2016.
Title: Depression and the Link with Cardiovascular Disease.

Authors: Dhar AK, , Barton DA.

Abstract: **This review provides an outline of the association between major depressive disorder (MDD) and coronary heart disease (CHD).** Much is known about the two individual clinical conditions; however, it is not until recently, biological mechanisms have been uncovered that link both MDD and CHD. The activation of stress pathways have been implicated as a neurochemical mechanism that links MDD and CHD. Depression is known to be associated with poorer outcomes of CHD. Psychological factors, such as major depression and stress, are now known as risk factors for developing CHD, which is as important and is independent of classic risk factors, such as hypertension, diabetes mellitus, and cigarette smoking. Both conditions have great socioeconomic importance given that depression and CHD are likely to be two of the three leading causes of global burden of disease. Better understanding of the common causal pathways will help us delineate more appropriate treatments.

Treatment of Diabetes: Major Historical Milestones

Weight Gain or Diabetes Could Be Just the Beginning of Your Problems

Source: Magy Onkol. 2006;50(2):127-35. Epub 2006 Aug 4.
Title: [Correlations of insulin resistance and neoplasms].
Authors: Suba Z, Ujpál M.
[Article in Hungarian]
Abstract: Insulin resistance is a worldwide risk factor for the two most dangerous human disease groups; namely, for cardiovascular lesions and malignancies. The insulin resistance syndrome have five basic criteria: hyperglycemia, visceral obesity, elevated serum triglyceride level, low HDL-cholesterol level (dyslipidemia) and hypertension. Each of these criteria alone are risk factors for cancer, and they mean together a multiple risk. Insulin resistance of the liver, skeletal muscles, and fatty tissue leads to a reactive hyperinsulinemia by the increased secretory activity of the beta-cells. Insulin has diverse metabolic effects, and at the same time is a growth factor. It enhances the production and mitogenic activity of other, insulin-like growth factors, and leads to pathological cell proliferation. In the uncompensated phase of insulin resistance hyperglycemia appears, which promotes tumorigenesis by several pathways. The elevated serum glucose level is advantageous for the increased DNA synthesis of the tumor cells. It provokes deliberation of free radicals, which will cause derangement of both the DNA and the enzymes having a

role in the repair mechanisms. Hyperglycemia leads to a nonenzymatic glycation of protein structures, and the glycated products enhance the deliberation of free radicals, cytokines and growth factors. Insulin resistance means an enhanced risk for breast, pancreas, liver, colon, bladder, prostate and oral cavity cancers. **The moderately increased fasting glucose level is also a risk factor for breast, stomach and colon cancers, even without manifestation of type 2 diabetes. Insulin resistance promotes tumor progression as well.** In cancer patients with hyperglycemia or type 2 diabetes, the rate of tumor recurrence, metastatic spread and fatal outcome is higher as compared with the tumor patients without metabolic disease. The correlation between insulin resistance and tumor promotion reveals new possibilities in the prevention and treatment of cancer. The healthy diet, physical activity and weight loss increase insulin sensitivity, and decrease the risk for both cardiovascular diseases and malignancies.

The Microbiota in Modern Man

Diabetes is one of the contributing causes of many of the top causes of death on the list of the Centers for Disease Control: heart disease, cancer, and stroke are all more likely when the person has diabetes. A diseased microbiota in the gut can lead to all kinds of negative health effects. See the FULLTEXT for a discussion of quinoa, a superfood.

FREE FULLTEXT
Source: Hepatobiliary Surg Nutr. 2012 Dec;1(1):25-52. doi: 10.3978/j.issn.2304-3881.2012.10.14.
Title: Nutrition of the critically ill - emphasis on liver and pancreas.
Author: Bengmark S
Abstract: About 25 million individuals undergo high risk surgery each year. Of these about 3 million will never return home from hospital, and the quality of life for many of those who return is often significantly impaired. Furthermore, many of those who manage to leave hospital have undergone severe life-threatening complications, mostly infections/sepsis. The development is strongly associated with the level of systemic inflammation in the body, which again is entirely a result of malfunctioning GI microbiota, a condition called dysbiosis, with deranged composition and function of the gastrointestinal microbiota from the mouth to the anus and impaired ability to maintain intact mucosal membrane functions and prevent leakage of toxins-bacterial endotoxins and whole or debris of bacteria, but also foods containing proteotoxins gluten, casein and zein and heat-induced molecules such as advanced glycation end products (AGEs) and advanced lipoxidation end products (ALEs). Markedly lower total anaerobic bacterial counts, particularly of the beneficial Bifidobacterium and Lactobacillus and higher counts of total facultative anaerobes such as Staphylococcus and Pseudomonas are often observed when analyzing the colonic microbiota. In addition Gram-negative facultative anaerobes are commonly identified microbial organisms in mesenteric lymph nodes and at serosal "scrapings" at laparotomy in patients suffering what is called "Systemic inflammation response system" (SIRS). Clearly the outcome is influenced by

preexisting conditions in those undergoing surgery, but not to the extent as one could expect. Several studies have for example been unable to find significant influence of pre-existing obesity. The outcome seems much more to be related to the lifestyle of the individual and her/his "maintenance" of the microbiota e.g., size and diversity of microbiota, normal microbiota, eubiosis, being highly preventive. About 75% of the food Westerners consume does not benefit microbiota in the lower gut. Most of it, refined carbohydrates, is already absorbed in the upper part of the GI tract, and of what reaches the large intestine is of limited value containing less minerals, less vitamins and other nutrients important for maintenance of the microbiota. The consequence is that the microbiota of modern man has a much reduced size and diversity in comparison to what our Paleolithic forefathers had, and individuals living a rural life have today. It is the artificial treatment provided by modern care, unfortunately often the only alternative, which belongs to the main contributor to poor outcome, among them; artificial ventilation, artificial nutrition, hygienic measures, use of skin penetrating devices, tubes and catheters, frequent use of pharmaceuticals, all known to significantly impair the total microbiome of the body and dramatically contribute to poor outcome. Attempts to reconstitute a normal microbiome have often failed as they have always been undertaken as a complement to and not an alternative to existing treatment schemes, especially treatments with antibiotics. **Modern nutrition formulas are clearly too artificial as they are based on mixture of a variety of chemicals, which alone or together induce inflammation. Alternative formulas, based on regular food ingredients, especially rich in raw fresh greens, vegetables and fruits and** with them healthy bacteria are suggested to be developed and tried.

Why Mom Made a Vinaigrette of Olive Oil and Vinegar for Your Daily Salad

Source: J Am Coll Cardiol. 2008 Jan 22;51(3):249-55. doi: 10.1016/j.jacc.2007.10.016.
Title: Dietary strategies for improving post-prandial glucose, lipids, inflammation, and cardiovascular health.
Authors: O'Keefe JH, Gheewala NM, O'Keefe JO.
Abstract: The highly processed, calorie-dense, nutrient-depleted diet favored in the current American culture frequently leads to exaggerated supraphysiological post-prandial spikes in blood glucose and lipids. This state, called post-prandial dysmetabolism, induces immediate oxidant stress, which increases in direct proportion to the increases in glucose and triglycerides after a meal. The transient increase in free radicals acutely triggers atherogenic changes including inflammation, endothelial dysfunction, hypercoagulability, and sympathetic hyperactivity. Post-prandial dysmetabolism is an independent predictor of future cardiovascular events even in nondiabetic individuals. **Improvements in diet exert profound and immediate favorable changes in the post-prandial dysmetabolism. Specifically, a diet high in minimally processed, high-fiber, plant-based foods such as vegetables and fruits, whole grains, legumes, and nuts will markedly blunt the post-meal increase in glucose, triglycerides, and inflam-**

mation. Additionally, lean protein, vinegar, fish oil, tea, cinnamon, calorie restriction, weight loss, exercise, and low-dose to moderate-dose alcohol each positively impact post-prandial dysmetabolism. Experimental and epidemiological studies indicate that eating patterns, such as the traditional Mediterranean or Okinawan diets, that incorporate these types of foods and beverages reduce inflammation and cardiovascular risk. This anti-inflammatory diet should be considered for the primary and secondary prevention of coronary artery disease and diabetes.

Top Recommendations for Dietary Change to Achieve Successful Weight-Loss and Natural Diabetes Control

First Know Thyself:
USDA Calculators for BMI, Nutritional Needs, and More:
https://fnic.nal.usda.gov/fnic/interactiveDRI/

Eat at Home to Lose Weight

FREE FULLTEXT
Source: Adolesc Health Med Ther. 2015 Jun 22;6:115-31. doi: 10.2147/AHMT.S37316. eCollection 2015.
Tite: Promoting family meals: a review of existing interventions and opportunities for future research.

Authors: Dwyer L, Oh A, Patrick H, Hennessy E.
Abstract: **Evidence suggests that regular family meals protect against unhealthy eating and obesity during childhood and adolescence.** However, there is limited information on ways to promote family meals as part of health promotion and obesity prevention efforts. The primary aim of this review was to synthesize the literature on strategies to promote family meals among families with school-aged children and adolescents. First, we reviewed interventions that assess family meals as an outcome and summarized strategies that have been used in these interventions. Second, we reviewed correlates and barriers to family meals to identify focal populations and target constructs for consideration in new interventions. During May 26-27, 2014, PubMed and PsycInfo databases were searched to identify literature on family meals published between January 1, 2000 and May 27, 2014. Two reviewers coded 2,115 titles/abstracts, yielding a sample of 139 articles for full-text review. Six interventions and 43 other studies presenting data on correlates of or barriers to family meals were included in the review. Four interventions resulted in greater family meal frequency. Although there were a small number of interventions, intervention settings were diverse and included the home, community, medical settings, the workplace, and the Internet. Common strategies were goal setting and interactive group activities, and intervention targets included cooking and food preparation, cost, shopping, and adolescent influence. Although methodological nuances may contribute to mixed findings, key correlates of family meals were employment, socioeconomic and demographic factors, family structure, and psychosocial constructs. Barriers to consider in future interventions include time and

scheduling challenges, cost, and food preferences. Increasing youth involvement in mealtime, tailoring interventions to family characteristics, and providing support for families experiencing time-related barriers are suggested strategies for future research.

List of Unprocessed Superfoods for Weight Loss

Processed foods fuel like hotdogs, ham, and Chef Boy R Dee can cause weight gain. In contrast, superfoods support weight loss. Looking for healthy options at the grocery store can sometimes feel like searching for a needle in a proverbial haystack. There are so many unhealthy, processed foods everywhere you look at the supermarket, it's no wonder that our country is facing an obesity epidemic. Add to this scenario our fixation on the Big Mac, large fries, and Diet Coke, and we really have a growing pandemic.

The good news is that, nutritious food is available, a partial list is found below. But, you say, you do not know how to cook? Luckily, I was a Columbia University Library Chief, so I know the best of the Web. If you want to look for great recipies by ingredients you have in your cupboard, I highly reccomend http://www.recipepuppy.com .

1. Almonds -Few superfoods deserve a spot on this list as much as almonds.
2. Apples- You've heard the expression, "An

apple a day keeps the doctor away".

3. Apricots- These orange-colored little fruits offer some great health benefits and are easy to snack on when you're on-the-go.
4. Artichokes - As long as you avoid drenching these fabulous green globes in mayo or butter, artichokes may actually help to lower your cholesterol.
5. Avocados - Avocados are pretty tough not to love. Not only do they pack quite a nutritional punch, they're incredibly satisfying, too!
6. Bananas - With their versatility and delicious taste, bananas may be one of the most pleasant ways to enhance your health.
7. Beans and Lentils - Beans and lentils provide a ton of fiber, protein, and a host of other health benefits.
8. Beets -You either love em' or hate em'. But if you love em', you'll have a leg up on those who don't.
9. Bell Peppers - Whether they're red, yellow, orange, or green, bell peppers pack quite a nutritional punch. Bake them, broil them, steam them, or eat them raw. Any way you slice them, bell peppers taste great!
10. Berries - For a fruit so small, berries are a true nutritional powerhouse!
11. Broccoli - When Mom told you to eat your broccoli, she knew what she was talking about!
12. Brussels Sprouts -Forget about the brussels sprouts you used to hide in your napkin as a kid. When prepared the right way, brussel sprouts are one of the tastiest veggies around. They're great for your health, too!
13. Cabbage -If you love cabbage, feel free to brag to those who don't about all of the health ben-

efits cabbage offers you.

14. Cantaloupe - This deliciously sweet melon is the perfect addition to a summer salad, and it can improve your health, too!

15. Carrots - Every kid knows that carrots are great for eyesight, but your vision isn't the only thing impacted by adding carrots to your diet.

16. Cauliflower - This cruciferous white veggie is tops in vitamin C and manganese and is excellent for your health.

17. Cherries - Cherries are one of those nutritional superfoods that you should devour while you have the chance. When cherry season arrives, you can feel good about what you're doing to preserve your brain and heart health. Cherries may be credited with slowing down the aging process and even with ending insomnia!

18. Chia Seeds - These tiny seeds are rich in Omega-3 fatty acids, and provide protein, healthy fats, and fiber.

19. Coconut - This tasty fruit is one of the most versatile superfoods out there.

20. Dark Chocolate -If you need a good excuse to eat your chocolate, look no further. Dark chocolate (not milk chocolate) may be great for cardiovascular health, premature aging and cancer. And guess what!? Dark chocolate is low on the glycemic index!

21. Eggs - Full of protein and extremely versatile, eggs are rich in nutrients. They can tackle a number of health problems and encourage weight loss.

22. Fish - While it's important to monitor which fish add nutritional value without any health

risks, if you can find the good stuff, you'll reap amazing benefits. Fish may protect your heart, fight cancer, and strengthen your immune system.

23. Flax Seeds - This little seed is a nutritional powerhouse. It may help your digestion, strengthen your immune system, and help with diabetes. The only seeds more powerful than flax are Chia seeds. But that doesn't mean you should forgo flax. It's far more readily available than Chia seeds are, and it is often more cost-effective for those on a budget.

24. Garlic - Most folks these days know the benefits of eating garlic. Aside from scaring vampires away, garlic may lower cholesterol, help with high blood pressure, fight against cancer, and even kill certain bacteria.

25. Grapes - This fruit is fabulously portable, so there's no excuse not to include grapes in your healthy eating plan. They may strengthen your eyes, help with circulation, and may even fight cancer and kidney stones.

26. Hot Peppers - Heat up your meals by adding hot peppers to your plate. They promise better digestion, an improved immune system, and better blood circulation and digestion. There is even a rumor that hot peppers aid in weight loss by increasing your metabolism

27. Kale - This superfood has powerful antioxidant qualities. Kale contains high amounts of phyto-chemicals that may help in preventing macular degeneration and cataracts. Kale may also help to combat many types of cancer, including breast cancer. Include this antioxidant powerhouse in your morning smoothie. Enjoy a SkinnyLicious Protein Smoothie for

breakfast or start your healthy eating lifestyle with a Cleanse & Detox Smoothie. Why go krazy for kale?

28. Kiwi -Kiwi is different from many other fruits because it contains a number of beneficial substances instead of just one or two. Kiwis are full of antioxidants and make you feel as if you're on a tropical vacation with every bite.

29. Lemons and Limes -These sour fruits are amazing at so many things. They may fight everything from cancer to the common cold. Never miss a chance to include these in your eating plan.

30. Low-Fat Yogurt and Kefir - Choose plain, non-fat Greek yogurt to pack protein on top of the numerous benefits including increased bone strength, lowered cholesterol, a stronger immune system, and better digestion. It may also be great for ulcers.

31. Mangoes - This tropical delight may help strengthen your memory as well as your digestion. It may also fight cancer and Alzheimer's disease.

32. Mushrooms - The lowly mushroom deserves to stand on a pedestal because of its medicinal uses. It may help control blood pressure and lower your cholesterol. And yes, like many other foods on this list, mushrooms may fight cancer, too!

33. Oats - Oats are well-known for their potential cholesterol-lowering abilities. But did you know they may also improve the condition of your skin and help fight diabetes?

34. Olive Oil - Olive oil can (and should!) be a part of many of your recipes. It may strengthen the heart, fight diabetes and cancer, and

can help with weight loss. For those with dry skin, it's an excellent way to cleanse your skin, as well! Just put a little oil on a cotton ball and wipe clean. You'll never use cleansers and water again!

35. Oranges - We all know that a nice glass of OJ goes well with just about any breakfast. But did you know that oranges may strengthen your immune system, fight cancer, and strengthen your heart?

36. Papaya - Papaya is a nutritional powerhouse. This yellow/orange fruit provides a number of health benefits and will leave your skin looking fabulous, too!

37. Peaches - These summertime treats are great for digestion and constipation.

38. Pineapple - Never miss a chance to eat pineapple! Not only is it absolutely delicious on a hot summer day, it may also strengthen your digestion, your bones, and can aid with weight loss.

39. Pumpkin - Some folks see pumpkins as something to carve once a year. But the truth is, your friendly jack-o'-lantern also provides tons of fiber and may control blood pressure and normalize heart function. So this year, carve your pumpkin a few hours before dark, and then bring in the flesh and seeds for cooking once the festivities are finished.

40. Pomegranates - These amazing fruits may have up to seven times the amount of antioxidants of green tea! Impressed? They may also fight cancer, reduce blood pressure, and lower bad cholesterol.

41. Quinoa - This "super grain" is high in fiber, filled with protein, and offers a pleasant nutty

flavor. It cooks up like rice and is naturally gluten-free. If you haven't tried it already, it's easy to prepare and surprisingly satisfying!

42. Spinach - Popeye had the right idea. You have to eat your spinach to grow strong! Why? Spinach may help fight cancer, improve your cardiovascular health, and improve brain function!

43. Spirulina - Don't let the idea of eating algae prevent you from enjoying all the benefits that spirulina has to offer. It is loaded with essential vitamins and nutrients. Toss it into a smoothie or add it to your favorite recipe, and you won't even know it's there.

44. Sprouts - Feasting on sprouts is a deliciously inexpensive way to reach total body nourishment. You'll be amazed at how many essential nutrients are packed into these tasty baby plants.

45. Sweet Potatoes - Healthy eaters know that sweet potatoes are a fantastic carb to include in your healthy eating plan! Why? Because they protect your vision, encourage a good mood, fight cancer, and keep your bones strong. That's why!

46. Tomatoes - These fabulous orbs may be big-time cancer fighters! They also help battle high cholesterol.

47. Walnuts - Easy to pack and snack on while out and about, nuts are loaded with healthy fats and offer a huge array of health benefits. Walnuts may be great for lowering cholesterol, fighting cancer and improving your memory.

48. Wild Caught Salmon - Wild caught salmon provides oodles of omega-3 essential fatty acids, a crucial bit of nutrition. But that's not

all. Salmon also provides many other vitamins like B3 and B12, which contribute to a healthy metabolism.

Fish Oil, Krill Oil and Diabetes

Want to reduce your risk of diabetes, disease, and overall inflammation of body and brain? Purified fish oil, cleaned of mercury, is an easy way to go. Also, wild sardines and salmon are good sources of Omega-3s which will reduce your risk of many diseases.

FREE FULLTEXT
Source: J Clin Med Res. 2015 Jan;7(1):8-12. doi: 10.14740/jocmr1964w. Epub 2014 Oct 16.
Title: Effects of intake of fish or fish oils on the development of diabetes.
Authors: Yanai H, Hamasaki H, Katsuyama H, Adachi H, Moriyama S, Sako A.
Abstract: The association between fish and fish oils intake and diabetes remains largely unknown. Here we systematically reviewed published articles (clinical trials, prospective cohort studies, systematic reviews and meta-analyses) about the effects of intake of fish or fish oils on the development of diabetes. An intake of fish oils seems not to affect insulin sensitivity, insulin secretion, beta-cell function or glucose tolerance. There is a considerable statistical heterogeneity in the overall summary estimates of the association between fish or fish oils consumption and the development of type 2 diabetes, which is partly explained by geographical differences. **Marine n-3 polyunsaturated fatty acids have beneficial effects on the prevention of type 2 diabetes in Asian populations.**

Source: Biomed Pharmacother. 1990;44(3):169-74.
Title: Fish oil: a panacea?

Authors: Bilo HJ, Gans RO.

Abstract: Since the first report by Bang and Dyerberg regarding the apparent beneficial effects of a fish oil-enriched diet on the incidence of atherosclerotic heart disease in Greenland eskimos, a considerable number of studies have been performed regarding the effects of omega-3 polyunsaturated fatty acids on the prevention and treatment of a variety of disease states not necessarily related to atherosclerosis. **Studies have been performed on healthy volunteers and in patients with hyperlipidaemia, atherosclerotic vascular disease, diabetes, asthma, psoriasis and chronic renal insufficiency, amongst others. Positive effects on platelet activity, lipid profile, blood rheology and blood pressure--all factors which are presumably of importance in the pathogenesis of atherosclerotic disease have been noted in these studies, albeit with a wide range of variability.** Some negative effects also appear to exist. However, some general conclusions can be made regarding the effects of a fish oil-enriched diet.

Krill Oil Versus Fish Oil

Source: Vasc Health Risk Manag. 2015 Aug 28;11:511-24. doi: 10.2147/VHRM.S85165. eCollection 2015.
Title: Comparison of bioavailability of krill oil versus fish oil and health effect.

Authors: Ulven SM, Holven KB.

Abstract: BACKGROUND:

The aim of this review is to summarize the effects of krill oil (KO) or fish oil (FO) on eicosapentaenoic acid (EPA) and docosahexaenoic acid (DHA) incorporation in plasma phospholipids or membrane of red blood cells (RBCs) as shown in human and animal studies. Furthermore, we discuss the findings in relation to the possible different health effects, focusing on lipids, inflammatory markers, cardiovascular disease risk, and biological functions of these two sources of long-chain n-3 polyunsaturated fatty acids (PUFAs).

METHODS: A literature search was conducted in PubMed in January 2015. In total, 113 articles were identified, but based on selection criteria, 14 original papers were included in the review.

RESULTS: Studies on bioavailability of EPA and DHA from KO and FO in humans and animals are limited and the interpretation is difficult, as different amounts of EPA and DHA have been used, duration of intervention differs, and different study groups have been included. Two human studies--one postprandial study and one intervention study--used the same amount of EPA and DHA from KO or FO, and they both showed that the bioavailability of EPA and DHA from KO seems to be higher than that from FO. Limited effects of KO and FO on lipids and inflammatory markers in human and animal studies were reported. Gene expression data from animal studies showed that FO upregulated the cholesterol synthesis pathway, which was the opposite of the effect mediated by KO. KO also regulated far more metabolic pathways than FO, which may indicate different biological effects of KO and FO.

CONCLUSION: **There seems to be a difference in bioavailability of EPA and DHA after intake of**

KO and FO, but more studies are needed before a firm conclusion can be made. It is also necessary to document the beneficial health effects of KO with more human studies and to elucidate if these effects differ from those after regular fish and FO intake.

Whey and Inflammation

Whey is not only for bodybuilders. The best whey to get is made from grass-fed, organic cow milk.

FREE FULLTEXT
Source: Lipids Health Dis. 2012 Jul 10;11:67. doi: 10.1186/1476-511X-11-67.
Title: Dietary whey protein lessens several risk factors for metabolic diseases: a review.
Authors: Sousa GT, Lira FS, Rosa JC, de Oliveira EP, Oyama LM, Santos RV, Pimentel GD.
Abstract: **Obesity and type 2 diabetes mellitus (DM) have grown in prevalence around the world, and recently, related diseases have been considered epidemic.** Given the high cost of treatment of obesity/DM-associated diseases, strategies such as dietary manipulation have been widely studied; among them, **the whey protein diet has reached popularity because it has been suggested as a strategy for the prevention and treatment of obesity and DM in both humans and animals.** Among its main actions, the following activities stand out: reduction of serum glucose in healthy individuals, impaired glucose tolerance in DM and obese patients; reduction in body weight; maintenance of muscle mass;

increases in the release of anorectic hormones such as cholecystokinin, leptin, and glucagon like-peptide 1 (GLP-1); and a decrease in the orexigenic hormone ghrelin. Furthermore, studies have shown that whey protein can also lead to reductions in blood pressure, inflammation, and oxidative stress.

Whey and Diabetes

Little Miss Muffet
Sat on her Tuffet
Eating her curds and whey.
Then came a spider,
Who sat down beside her,
And scared Miss Muffet away.
Whey was more common in our diet hundreds of years ago, as can be seen from the above Mother Goose nursery rhyme. What is whey protein anyway? Typically, it is the stuff left over after cheeses are made. Whey has been popular with bodybuilders for a long time, as it helps nourish the muscles, so they can add muscle mass more easily, and it is good for the waist..

Finally, whey is a precursor of the "master antioxidant" glutathione, in the brain and body, in adding to its long list of positive effects. Whey is probably one of the easiest and effective foodstuffs to add to the diet. The best form of whey to get for these many benefits is whey from grass-fed cows that is cold processed, so the unique beneficial properties of the whey are not lost. It is possible to make whey at home, but it is easier to buy it.

Source: Diabetologia. 2014 Sep;57(9):1807-11. doi:
10.1007/s00125-014-3305-x. Epub 2014 Jul 10.
Title: Incretin, insulinotropic and glucose-lowering
effects of whey protein pre-load in type 2 diabetes: a
randomised clinical trial.
Authors: Jakubowicz D, Froy O, Ahrén B, Boaz M,
Landau Z, Bar-Dayan Y, Ganz T, Barnea M, Wain-
stein J.
Abstract: AIMS/HYPOTHESIS: Since protein
ingestion is known to stimulate the secretion of
glucagon-like peptide-1 (GLP-1), we hypothesised
that enhancing GLP-1 secretion to harness its insu-
linotropic/beta cell-stimulating activity with whey
protein pre-load may have beneficial glucose-lowering effects in type 2 diabetes. **METHODS:** In a
randomised, open-label crossover clinical trial, we
studied 15 individuals with well-controlled type 2
diabetes who were not taking any medications except
for sulfonylurea or metformin. These participants
consumed, on two separate days, 50 g whey in 250
ml water or placebo (250 ml water) followed by a
standardised high-glycaemic-index breakfast in a
hospital setting. Participants were randomised using a coin flip. The primary endpoints of the study
were plasma concentrations of glucose, intact GLP-1
and insulin during the 30 min following meal ingestion. **RESULTS:** In each group, 15 patients were
analysed. The results showed that over the whole 180
min post-meal period, glucose levels were reduced by
28% after whey pre-load with a uniform reduction
during both early and late phases. Insulin and C-
peptide responses were both significantly higher (by
105% and 43%, respectively) with whey pre-load.
Notably, the early insulin response was 96% higher
after whey. Similarly, both total GLP-1 (tGLP-1)
and intact GLP-1 (iGLP-1) levels were significantly

higher (by 141% and 298%, respectively) with whey pre-load. Dipeptidyl peptidase 4 plasma activity did not display any significant difference after breakfast between the groups. **CONCLUSIONS / INTERPRETATION:** In summary, consumption of whey protein shortly before a high-glycaemic-index breakfast increased the early prandial and late insulin secretion, augmented tGLP-1 and iGLP-1 responses and reduced postprandial glycaemia in type 2 diabetic patients. **Whey protein may therefore represent a novel approach for enhancing glucose-lowering strategies in type 2 diabetes.**

Magnesium- It's good for what ails you

More than three hundred enzymatic systems in the body require magnesium, yet about half of Americans do not get an adequate amount of magnesium in their diets. However, excess magnesium can be toxic. When supplementing with magnesium, it is generally accepted to take the magnesium and calcium it at night in a 2:1 ratio- calcium to magnesium, as a sleep aid as well as to keep the minerals balanced. You can also supplement with proper amounts of Vitamin D, C, B6, B12, Folic Acid, Selenium, Chromium, Iron, and B5 so the magnesium works better. These nutrients work in synergy with the magnesium and calcium and are anti-inflammatory. Even if you are taking a multivitamin, you probably are not getting enough magnesium. Most multivitamins give you 100% of manganese, which can easily be confused with magnesium. Remember to take no more than the RDA, Recommended Daily Allowance of any nutraceutical. Read the labels to make sure you are doing the supplementation correctly and the appropriate doses- more does not necessarily equal better.

FREE FULLTEXT
Source: Rocz Panstw Zakl Hig. 2013;64(3):165-71.
Title: Magnesium: its role in nutrition and carcinogenesis.
Authors: Blaszczyk U, Duda-Chodak A.

Abstract: Magnesium (Mg^{2+}) plays a key role in many essential cellular processes such as intermediary metabolism, DNA replication and repair, transporting potassium and calcium ions, cell proliferation together with signalling transduction. Dietary sources rich in magnesium are whole and unrefined grains, seeds, cocoa, nuts, almonds and green leafy vegetables. Hard water is also considered to be an important source of magnesium beneficial to human health. The daily dietary intake of magnesium is however frequently found to be below that recommended in Western countries. **Indeed, it is recognised that magnesium deficiency may lead to many disorders of the human body, where for instance magnesium depletion is believed to play an important role in the aetiology of the following; cardiovascular disease (including thrombosis, atherosclerosis, ischemic heart disease, myocardial infarction, hypertension, arrhythmias and congestive heart failure in human), as well as diabetes mellitus, gastrointestinal (GI) tract disease, liver cirrhosis and diseases of the thyroid and parathyroid glands.** Insufficient dietary intake of magnesium may also significantly affect the development and exacerbation of ADHD (Attention Deficit- Hyperactivity Disorder) symptoms in children. The known links between magnesium and carcinogenesis still remain unclear and complex, with conflicting results being reported from many experimental, epidemiological and clinical studies; further knowledge is thus required. Mg2+ ions are enzyme cofactors involved in DNA repair mechanisms that maintain genomic stability and fidelity. Any magnesium deficiencies could thereby cause a dysfunction of these systems to occur leading to DNA mutations. Magnesium deficiency may also be associated with inflammation and increased levels of free radicals where both inflammatory mediators and free radicals so arising could cause oxidative DNA damage and therefore tumour formation. The presented review article now provides a summary discussion of the various research performed concerning the impact that low magnesium intake has on tumour incidence; this includes impairment of magnesium homeostasis frequently observed in tumour cells, the influence of magnesium depletion on the progression of existing tumours and the occurrence of hypo-magnesaemia when patients are treated with certain anticancer drugs.

A Mix of Helpful Nutrients- And an Insulin Mimetic

Niacin, Chromium and Glutathione affect Glucose Tolerance Factor, which is necessary for insulin to func-

tion optimally. Niacin-bound chromium has been demonstrated to be more bioavailable than chromium picolinate and more efficacious while no toxicity has been reported, when taken at recommended levels. GTF is depleted by sugar and alcohol, so a lot of people start having blood sugar problems by the time they reach forty. Although there are a plethora of other reasons for Type II Diabetes, many with a blood sugar problem is low on GTF.

Replenishing your GTF is a good idea for long term health. Whey protein converts to the most powerful anti-oxidant Glutathione. Alternatively, N-Acetylcysteine otherwise known to many as *NAC also works to raise Glutathione levels for many people. The hard part in making GTF seems to be linking the Niacin to Chromium. It can take people several months to improve their GTF if they use Chromium Picolinate instead of Niacin bound Chromium. Vanadium has Insulin like properties. A fountain in Japan rich in Vanadium is popular with diabetics. No one is certain how it works.*

Supplements made from Brewer's Yeast such as selenium contain the end product GTF. This can help with appetite control. When someone's Insulin is not functioning properly, losing weight is very difficult because cells do not get a chance to use all the Glucose they want, and instead, your liver converts the excess Glucose in your blood to fat. Glucose in high quantities is toxic, and rots your arteries and nerves in a process called glycation. It is best to discuss everything with your doctor, but his training is to give you a pancreatic stimulant to squeeze out more Insulin instead of shoring up GTF. The Biochemistry of GTF was discovered by the U.S. Dept. of Agriculture.

Source: Altern Med Rev. 2009 Jun;14(2):177-80.
Title: Vanadium (vanadyl sulfate). Monograph.

From monograph: *"Seven type 2 diabetic subjects were given oral doses of [Vanadium] BEOV (AKP-020), 20 mg daily for 28 days. Researchers observed reductions in fasting blood glucose and hemoglobin A1c (HbA1c), and improved responses to oral glucose tolerance testing, compared to exacerbated diabetic symptoms in the two placebo controls.*

Drug-Nutrient Interactions: Anticoagulant/Anti-platelet Drugs *In vitro studies of sodium orthovanadate (vanadate) demonstrated prolonged clotting time, which was additive in the presence of heparin. This suggests the vanadate form of vanadium may potentiate anticoagulant therapy when administered concurrently.24* ***Antidiabetic Drugs*** *Concurrent use of vanadyl sulfate with insulin or oral hypoglycemic agents for diabetes may have an additive effect, as vanadyl sulfate can increase insulin sensitivity in individuals with type 2 diabetes.17-19* ***Side Effects and Toxicity*** *Mild gastrointestinal discomfort in the form of abdominal cramps and loose stools has been reported with ingestion of vanadyl sulfate at therapeutic doses.17 Toxicity studies on rats concluded vanadyl sulfate, in doses necessary to cause euglycemia, was not toxic after one year of administration; however, vanadium may be retained in organs for months after conclusion of administration.25 Acute vanadium toxicity has not been observed in humans. In rats, acute poisoning from sodium vanadate resulted in enteritis, mild liver congestion, and slight renal tubule degeneration.26* ***Dosage*** *There is no RDA for vanadium. A daily intake of 10-100 mcg is considered safe and adequate from food sources. The average diet supplies between 6-18 mcg of vanadium daily. A therapeutic dosage for management of type 2 diabetes is at least*

*50 mg vanadyl sulfate twice daily. 17-19 **Warnings and Contraindications** Caution should be used when combining vanadium supplements with any blood-sugar lowering medication as the combination may induce hypoglycemia."*

Fiber, Weight Loss, and Diabetes Control

Metamucil works for this, Citrucel does not confer the same benefits.

Source: Food Funct. 2016 Feb 29. [Epub ahead of print]
Title: Dietary fiber and blood pressure control.
Authors: Aleixandre A, Miguel M.

Abstract: In the past few years, new strategies to control blood pressure levels are emerging by developing new bioactive components of foods. Fiber has been linked to the prevention of a number of cardiovascular diseases and disorders. ☒-Glucan, the main soluble fiber component in oat grains, was initially linked to a reduction in plasma cholesterol. **Several studies have shown afterward that dietary fiber may also improve glycaemia, insulin resistance and weight loss.** The effect of dietary fiber on arterial blood pressure has been the subject of far fewer studies than its effect on the above-mentioned variables, but research has already shown that fiber intake can decrease arterial blood pressure in hypertensive rats. Moreover, certain fibers can improve arterial blood pressure when administered to hypertensive and pre-hypertensive subjects. The present review summarizes all those studies which attempt to establish the antihypertensive effects of dietary fiber, as well as its effect on other cardiovascular risk factors.

World Cuisines and Traditional Styles of Healthy Eating

The Hunter-Gatherer Diet- The Good Old Days

Green is Good

FREE FULLTEXT
Source: Appetite. 2014 Oct;81:295-304. doi: 10.1016/j.appet.2014.06.101. Epub 2014 Jun 30.
Title: Body weight loss, reduced urge for palatable food and increased release of GLP-1 through daily supplementation with green-plant membranes for three months in overweight women.
Authors: Montelius C, Erlandsson D, Vitija E, Stenblom EL, Egecioglu E, Erlanson-Albertsson C.
Abstract: The frequency of obesity has risen dramatically in recent years but only few effective and safe drugs are available. We investigated if green-plant membranes, previously shown to reduce subjective hunger and promote satiety signals, could affect body weight when given long-term. 38 women (40-65 years of age, body mass index 25-33 kg/m(2)) were randomized to dietary supplementation with either green-plant membranes (5 g) or placebo, con-

sumed once daily before breakfast for 12 weeks. All individuals were instructed to follow a three-meal paradigm without any snacking between the meals and to increase their physical activity. Body weight change was analysed every third week as was blood glucose and various lipid parameters. On days 1 and 90, following intake of a standardized breakfast, glucose, insulin and glucagon-like peptide 1 (GLP-1) in plasma were measured, as well as subjective ratings of hunger, satiety and urge for different palatable foods, using visual analogue scales. Subjects receiving green-plant membranes lost significantly more body weight than did those on placebo ($p < 0.01$). Mean weight loss with green-plant extract was 5.0 ± 2.3 kg compared to 3.5 ± 2.3 kg in the control group. Consumption of green-plant membranes also reduced total and LDL-cholesterol ($p < 0.01$ and $p < 0.05$ respectively) compared to control. Single-meal tests performed on day 1 and day 90 demonstrated an increased postprandial release of GLP-1 and decreased urge for sweet and chocolate on both occasions in individuals supplemented with green-plant membranes compared to control. Waist circumference, body fat and leptin decreased in both groups over the course of the study, however there were no differences between the groups. **In conclusion, addition of green-plant membranes as a dietary supplement once daily induces weight loss, improves obesity-related risk-factors, and reduces the urge for palatable food. The mechanism may reside in the observed increased release of GLP-1.**

Organic Veggies are Richer in Nutrients

Source: Int J Environ Res Public Health. 2014 Apr 8;11(4):3870-93. doi: 10.3390/ijerph110403870.
Title: Contribution of organically grown crops to human health.

Authors: Johansson E, Hussain A, Kuktaite R, Andersson SC, Olsson ME.

Abstract: An increasing interest in organic agriculture for food production is seen throughout the world and one key reason for this interest is the assumption that organic food consumption is beneficial to public health. The present paper focuses on the background of organic agriculture, important public health related compounds from crop food and variations in the amount of health related compounds in crops. In addition, influence of organic farming on health related compounds, on pesticide residues and heavy metals in crops, and relations between organic food and health biomarkers as well as in vitro studies are also the focus of the present paper. Nutritionally beneficial compounds of highest relevance for public health were micronutrients, especially Fe and Zn, and bioactive compounds such as carotenoids (including pro-vitamin A compounds), tocopherols (including vitamin E) and phenolic compounds. Extremely large variations in the contents of these compounds were seen, depending on genotype, climate, environment, farming conditions, harvest time, and part of the crop. Highest amounts seen were related to the choice of genotype and were also increased by genetic modification of the crop. Organic cultivation did not influence the content of most of the nutritionally beneficial compounds, except the phenolic compounds that were increased with the amounts of pathogens. However, higher amounts of pesticide residues and in many cases also of heavy metals were seen in the conventionally produced crops compared to the organic ones. Animal studies as well as in vitro studies showed a clear indication of a beneficial effect of organic food/extracts as compared to conventional ones. **Thus, consumption of organic food seems to be positive from a public health point of view, although the reasons are unclear, and synergistic effects between various constituents within the food are likely.**

Meat Raised Without Antibiotics or Hormones

FREE FULLTEXT
Source: Toxicol Res. 2010 Dec;26(4):301-13. doi: 10.5487/TR.2010.26.4.301.
Title: Risk assessment of growth hormones and antimicrobial residues in meat.

Abstract: Growth promoters including hormonal substances and antibiotics are used legally and illegally in food producing animals for the growth promotion of livestock animals. Hormonal substances still under debate in terms of their human health impacts are estradiol-17, progesterone, testosterone, zeranol, trenbolone, and melengestrol acetate (MGA) . Many of the risk assessment results of natural steroid hormones have presented negligible impacts when they are used under good veterinary practices. For synthetic hormonelike substances, ADIs and MRLs have been established for food safety along with the approval of animal treatment. Small amounts of antibiotics added to feedstuff present growth promotion effects via the prevention of infectious diseases at doses lower than therapeutic dose. The induction of antimicrobial resistant bacteria and the disruption of normal human intestinal flora are major concerns in terms of human health impact. Regulatory guidance such as ADIs and MRLs fully reflect the impact on human gastrointestinal microflora. However, before deciding on any risk management options, risk assessments of antimicrobial resistance require large-scale evidence regarding the relationship between antimicrobial use in food-producing animals and the occurrence of antimicrobial resistance in human pathogens. **In this article, the risk profiles of hormonal and antibacterial growth promoters are provided based on recent toxicity and human exposure information, and recommendations for risk management to prevent human health impacts by the use of growth promoters are also presented.**

Locally Grown Foodstuffs are Best

FREE FULLTEXT
Source: Am J Clin Nutr. 2014 May;99(5):1117-25. doi: 10.3945/ajcn.113.066746. Epub 2014 Mar 26.
Title: The New Nordic Diet is an effective tool in environmental protection: it reduces the associated socioeconomic cost of diets.
Author: Saxe H.
Abstract: BACKGROUND: The New Nordic Diet

(NND) was designed by gastronomic, nutritional, and environmental specialists to be a palatable, healthy, and sustainable diet containing 35% less meat than the Average Danish Diet (ADD); more whole-grain products, nuts, fruit, and vegetables; locally grown food in season; and >75% organic produce. The environmental impact of the 2 diets was compared based on 16 impact categories, which were monetized to evaluate the overall socioeconomic effect of a shift from an ADD to an NND. OBJECTIVE: The objective was to determine whether this diet shift can be an effective tool in environmental protection. DESIGN: The 3 features by which this diet shift affects the environment-composition, transport (import), and type of production (organic/conventional)-were separately investigated by using life cycle assessment. RESULTS: When both diet composition and transport were taken into account, the NND reduced the environmental impact relative to the ADD measured by all 16 impact categories. The socio-economic savings related to this diet shift was €266/person per year, or 32% of the overall environmental cost of the ADD. When the actual 8% content of organic produce in the ADD and the 84% content of organic produce in the investigated recipe-based NND were also taken into account, the NND reduced the environmental impact relative to the ADD measured by only 10 of the 16 impact categories whereas 6 were increased. The socio-economic savings related to the diet shift were lowered to €42/person per year, or 5% of the overall environmental cost of the ADD. CONCLUSION: **Reducing the content of meat and excluding most long-distance imports were of substantial environmental and socioeconomic advantage to the NND when compared with the ADD, whereas including high amounts of organic produce was a disadvantage.**

Berries and Health

FREE FULLTEXT
Source: Rocz Panstw Zakl Hig. 2014;65(2):79-85.
Title: Flavonoids--food sources and health benefits.
Authors: Kozłowska A, Szostak-Wegierek D.
Abstract: **Flavonoids are a group of bioactive compounds that are extensively found in foodstuffs of plant origin. Their regular consumption is associated with reduced risk of a number of chronic diseases, including cancer, cardiovascular disease (CVD) and neurodegenerative disorders.** Flavonoids are classified into subgroups based on their chemical structure: flavanones, flavones, flavonols, flavan-3-ols, anthocyanins and isoflavones. Their actions at the molecular level include antioxidant effects, as well the ability to modulate several key enzymatic pathways. The growing body of scientific evidence indicates that flavonoids play a beneficial role in disease prevention, however further clinical and epidemiological trials are greatly needed. Among dietary sources of flavonoids there are fruits, vegetables, nuts, seeds and spices. Consumption of these substances with diet appears to be safe. It seems that a diet rich in flavonoids is beneficial and its promotion is thus justifiable.

Nuts about Nuts

Nuts and Inflammation

It's common knowledge that in moderation, nuts are good for the health. Here is why.

Source: Nutrients. 2010 Jul;2(7):652-82. doi:
10.3390/nu2070683. Epub 2010 Jun 24.

Title: Health benefits of nut consumption.

Author: Ros E.

Abstract: Nuts (tree nuts and peanuts) are nutrient
dense foods with complex matrices rich in unsaturat-
ed fatty and other bioactive compounds: high-quality
vegetable protein, fiber, minerals, tocopherols, phytosterols, and phenolic compounds. By virtue of
their unique composition, nuts are likely to benefi-
cially impact health outcomes. Epidemiologic studies have associated nut consumption with a reduced
incidence of coronary heart disease and gallstones in
both genders and diabetes in women. Limited evidence also suggests beneficial effects on hypertension,
cancer, and inflammation. Interventional studies
consistently show that nut intake has a cholesterol-
lowering effect, even in the context of healthy diets,
and there is emerging evidence of beneficial effects
on oxidative stress, inflammation, and vascular re-
activity. Blood pressure, visceral adiposity and the
metabolic syndrome also appear to be positively
influenced by nut consumption. **Thus it is clear that
nuts have a beneficial impact on many cardiovascular risk factors. Contrary to expectations, epidemiologic studies and clinical trials suggest that
regular nut consumption is unlikely to contribute
to obesity and may even help in weight loss.** Safety
concerns are limited to the infrequent occurrence of
nut allergy in children. In conclusion, nuts are nutrient rich foods with wide-ranging cardiovascular and
metabolic benefits, which can be readily incorporated
into healthy diets.

FREE FULLTEXT
Source: Am J Clin Nutr. 2014 Jul;100 Suppl 1:412S-22S. doi: 10.3945/ajcn.113.071456. Epub 2014 Jun 11.
Title: A review of the effects of nuts on appetite, food intake, metabolism, and body weight.

Authors: Tan SY, Dhillon J, Mattes RD.

Abstract: Tree nuts and peanuts are good sources of many nutrients and antioxidants, but they are also energy dense. The latter often limits intake because of concerns about their possible contribution to positive energy balance. However, evidence to date suggests that nuts are not associated with predicted weight gain. **This is largely due to their high satiety value, leading to strong compensatory dietary responses, inefficiency in absorption of the energy they contain, a possible increment in resting energy expenditure, and an augmentation of fat oxidation.** Preliminary evidence suggests that these properties are especially evident when they are consumed as snacks.

Coconut: The All-Giving Tree

FREE FULLTEXT
Source: Asian Pac J Trop Med. 2011 Mar;4(3):241-7. doi: 10.1016/S1995-7645(11)60078-3. Epub 2011 Apr 12.
Title: Coconut (Cocos nucifera L.: Arecaceae): in health promotion and disease prevention.

Authors: DebMandal M, Mandal S.

Abstract: Coconut, Cocos nucifera L., is a tree that is cultivated for its multiple utilities, mainly for its nutritional and medicinal values. The various products of coconut include tender coconut water, copra, coconut oil, raw kernel, coconut cake, coconut toddy, coconut shell and wood based products, coconut leaves, coir pith etc. Its all parts are used in someway or another in the daily life of the people in the traditional coconut growing areas. It is the unique source of various natural products for the development of medicines against various diseases and also for the development of industrial products. **The parts of its fruit like coconut kernel and tender coconut water have numerous medicinal properties such as antibacterial, antifungal, antiviral, antiparasitic, antidermatophytic, antioxidant, hypoglycemic, hepatoprotective, immunostimulant. Coconut water and coconut kernel contain microminerals and nutrients, which are essential to human health, and hence coconut is used as food by the peoples in the globe, mainly in the tropical countries.** The coconut palm is, therefore, eulogised as 'Kalpavriksha' (the all giving tree) in Indian classics, and thus the current review describes the facts and phenomena related to its use in health and disease prevention.

The Mediterranean Diet

The Mediterranean diets are rich in fish, fruit, and antioxidants. These diets reduce inflammation and disease across many markers of disease. They reduce weight gain, and they are good for the heart.

The Biblical and Middle Eastern Roots of the Mediterranean Diet

FREE FULLTEXT
Source: Public Health Nutr. 2011
Dec;14(12A):2288-95. doi: 10.1017/
S1368980011002539.
Title: The Middle Eastern and biblical origins of the
Mediterranean diet.
Authors: Berry EM1, Arnoni Y, Aviram M.
Abstract: OBJECTIVE: To place the Mediterranean
diet (MedDi) in the context of the cultural history
of the Middle East and emphasise the health effects
of some of the biblical seven species - wheat, barley,
grapes, figs, pomegranates, olives and date honey.
DESIGN: Review of the literature concerning the
benefits of these foods.
SETTING: Middle East and Mediterranean Basin.
SUBJECTS: Mediterranean populations and clinical
studies utilising the MedDi.
RESULTS AND CONCLUSIONS: The MedDi has
been associated with lower rates of CVD, and epidemiological evidence promotes the benefits of consuming fruit and vegetables. Recommended foods
for optimal health include whole grain, fish, wine,
pomegranates, figs, walnuts and extra virgin olive
oil. The biblical traditional diet, including the seven
species and additional Mediterranean fruits, has great
health advantages, especially for CVD. In addition
to the diet, lifestyle adaptation that involves increasing physical activity and organised meals, together
with healthy food choices, is consistent with the
traditional MedDi. **The MedDi is a manageable,
lifestyle-friendly diet that, when fortified with its
biblical antecedent attributes, may prove to be
even more enjoyable and considerably healthier**

in combating the obesogenic environment and in decreasing the risks of the non-communicable diseases of modern life than conventional, modern dietary recommendations. The biblical seven species, together with other indigenous foods from the Middle East, are now scientifically recognised as healthy foods, and further improve the many beneficial effects of the MedDi.

MediterrAsian Diet

Source: Oxid Med Cell Longev. 2013;2013:707421. doi: 10.1155/2013/707421. Epub 2013 Aug 28.
Title: Nutrition and healthy ageing: calorie restriction or polyphenol-rich "MediterrAsian" diet?
Authors: Pallauf K, Giller K, Huebbe P, Rimbach G.
Abstract: **Diet plays an important role in mammalian health and the prevention of chronic diseases such as cardiovascular disease (CVD).** Incidence of CVD is low in many parts of Asia (e.g., Japan) and the Mediterranean area (e.g., Italy, Spain, Greece, and Turkey). The Asian and the Mediterranean diets are rich in fruit and vegetables, thereby providing high amounts of plant bioactives including polyphenols, glucosinolates, and antioxidant vitamins. Furthermore, oily fish which is rich in omega-3 fatty acids is an important part of the Asian (e.g., Japanese) and also of the Mediterranean diets. There are specific plant bioactives which predominantly occur in the Mediterranean (e.g., resveratrol from red wine, hydroxytyrosol, and oleuropein from olive oil) and

in the Asian diets (e.g., isoflavones from soybean and epigallocatechin gallate from green tea). Interestingly, when compared to calorie restriction which has been repeatedly shown to increase healthspan, these polyphenols activate similar molecular targets such as Sirt1. We suggest that a so-called "MediterrAsian" diet combining sirtuin-activating foods (= sirtfoods) of the Asian as well as Mediterranean diet may be a promising dietary strategy in preventing chronic diseases, thereby ensuring health and healthy ageing. Future (human) studies are needed which take the concept suggested here of the MediterrAsian diet into account.

The Mediterranean diet is great for keeping a healthy weight

Not only does the Mediterranean diet taste good, it's good for you!

Source: Nutrición hospitalaria: organo oficial de la Sociedad Española de Nutrición Parenteral y Enteral. Jan-Feb 2010..
Title: Behavioural therapy in the treatment of obesity (II): role of the Mediterranean diet.

Abstract: Objectives: Obesity is the consequence of an imbalance between energy intake and expenditure, food intake being affected by multiple factors -psychological, social, work-related, etc. This revision discusses the role of diet in the behavioural treatment (BT) of obesity, which faces multiple approaches and focuses on patients' behaviour rather than their mere energy intake.

Setting: Recent literature has been revised that deals with the health benefits of Mediterranean diet in order to assess its suitability for obesity treatment based on BT.

Results: BT helps patients to develop skills and techniques in order to adopt proper habits and attain their healthiest weight. Patients learn to establish realistic goals, both as regards weight and behaviour, and to evaluate their progress in modifying eating and exercising habits. The application of the Mediterranean diet in obesity treatment presents various advantages which are based on the principles of this diet -wide variety of food, high carbohydrate content, or high satiating capacity, which prevents specific hunger and ketogenesis-, and has been demonstrated to be effective in reducing body weight.

Conclusions: BT based on the Mediterranean diet is a useful tool for obesity treatment. The Mediterranean diet provides the patients with a diet established on widely recognised nutritional benefits, suitable to their social and daily life, and that can be easily followed in the long term, according to the objectives of BT. *For these reasons, Mediterranean diet-based BT helps to prolong both the treatment and maintenance periods and therefore contributes to a more stable weight loss.*

Olive Oil and Inflammation

Olive oil is a great addition to any diet due to its anti-inflammatory profile.

Source: Pharmacol Rev. 2000 Dec;52(4):673-751.
Title: The effects of plant flavonoids on mammalian cells: implications for inflammation, heart disease, and cancer.

Authors: Middleton E Jr, Kandaswami C, Theoharides TC.

Abstract: Flavonoids are nearly ubiquitous in plants and are recognized as the pigments responsible for the colors of leaves, especially in autumn. They are rich in seeds, citrus fruits, olive oil, tea, and red wine. They are low molecular weight compounds composed of a three-ring structure with various substitutions. This basic structure is shared by tocopherols (vitamin E). Flavonoids can be subdivided according to the presence of an oxy group at position 4, a double bond between carbon atoms 2 and 3, or a hydroxyl group in position 3 of the C (middle) ring. These characteristics appear to also be required for best activity, especially antioxidant and antiproliferative, in the systems studied. The particular hydroxylation pattern of the B ring of the flavonoids increases their activities, especially in inhibition of mast cell secretion. Certain plants and spices containing flavonoids have been used for thousands of years in traditional Eastern medicine. **In spite of the voluminous literature available, however, Western medicine has not yet used flavonoids therapeutically, even though their safety record is exceptional. Suggestions are made where such possibilities may be worth pursuing.**

The Mediterranean Diet: On the Genomic Level

FREE FULLTEXT
Source: Nutrients. 2016 Apr 13;8(4). pii: E218. doi: 10.3390/nu8040218.
Title: Nutritional Genomics and the Mediterranean Diet's Effects on Human Cardiovascular Health.

Authors: Fitó M1, Konstantinidou V2.

Abstract: The synergies and cumulative effects among different foods and nutrients are what produce the benefits of a healthy dietary pattern. Diets and dietary patterns are a major environmental factor that we are exposed to several times a day. People can learn how to control this behavior in order to promote healthy living and aging, and to prevent diet-related diseases. **To date, the traditional Mediterranean diet has been the only well-studied pattern. Stroke incidence, a number of classical risk factors including lipid profile and glycaemia, emergent risk factors such as the length of telomeres, and emotional eating behavior can be affected by genetic predisposition.** Adherence to the Mediterranean diet could exert beneficial effects on these risk factors. Our individual genetic make-up should be taken into account to better prevent these traits and their subsequent consequences in cardiovascular disease development. In the present work, we review the results of nutritional genomics explaining the role of the Mediterranean diet in human cardiovascular disease. A multidisciplinary approach is necessary to extract knowledge from large-scale data.

The Asian Diet and Maintaining a Healthy Weight

For years people have noticed how thin and beautiful many people from Asia are. It turns out that it is not just their genetics that causes them to be healthy. A big part of their apparent thinness and health of Asians is due to their traditional diet. A diet rich in fish, vegetables, seaweed, green tea, fish sauce (which contains some vinegar), garlic, onion, ginger, curry. with much bicycling and and walking thrown in is bound to be good for the health. The following articles show the health benefits of many of these traditional components of the Asian way of life.

Green Tea and Weight Loss

Source: American Journal of Clinical Nutrition. Jan 2010.
Title: Effect of green tea catechins with or without caffeine on anthropometric measures: a systematic review and meta-analysis.
Authors: Phung OJ, Baker WL, Matthews LJ, Lanosa M, Thorne A, Coleman CI.

Abstract: Background: Green tea catechins (GTCs) with or without caffeine have been studied in randomized controlled trials (RCTs) for their effect on anthropometric measures and have yielded conflicting results.
Objective: The objective was to perform a systematic review and meta-analysis of RCTs of GTCs on anthropometric variables, including body mass index

(BMI), body weight, waist circumference (WC), and waist-to-hip ratio (WHR).

DESIGN: A systematic literature search of MED-LINE, EMBASE, CENTRAL, and the Natural Medicines Comprehensive Database was conducted through April 2009. RCTs that evaluated GTCs with or without caffeine and that reported BMI, body weight, WC, or WHR were included. The weighted mean difference of change from baseline (with 95% CIs) was calculated by using a random-effects model. Results: Fifteen studies (n = 1243 patients) met the inclusion criteria. On meta-analysis, GTCs with caffeine decreased BMI (-0.55; 95% CI: -0.65, -0.40), body weight (-1.38 kg; 95% CI: -1.70, -1.06), and WC (-1.93 cm; 95% CI: -2.82, -1.04) but not WHR compared with caffeine alone. GTC ingestion with caffeine also significantly decreased body weight (-0.44 kg; 95% CI: -0.72, -0.15) when compared with a caffeine-free control. Studies that evaluated GTCs without concomitant caffeine administration did not show benefits on any of the assessed anthropometric endpoints.
Conclusions: **The administration of GTCs with caffeine is associated with statistically significant reductions in BMI, body weight, and WC; however, the clinical significance of these reductions is modest at best. Current data do not suggest that GTCs alone positively alter anthropometric measurement.**

FREE FULLTEXT
Source: Journal of the American College of Cardiology. Jan 22 2008.
Title: Dietary strategies for improving post-prandial glucose, lipids, inflammation, and cardiovascular

health.

Authors: O'Keefe JH, Gheewala NM, O'Keefe JO.

Abstract The highly processed, calorie-dense, nutrient-depleted diet favored in the current American culture frequently leads to exaggerated supraphysiological post-prandial spikes in blood glucose and lipids. This state, called post-prandial dysmetabolism, induces immediate oxidant stress, which increases in direct proportion to the increases in glucose and triglycerides after a meal. The transient increase in free radicals acutely triggers atherogenic changes including inflammation, endothelial dysfunction, hypercoagulability, and sympathetic hyperactivity. Post-prandial dysmetabolism is an independent predictor of future cardiovascular events even in nondiabetic individuals. Improvements in diet exert profound and immediate favorable changes in the post-prandial dysmetabolism. **Specifically, a diet high in minimally processed, high-fiber, plant-based foods such as vegetables and fruits, whole grains, legumes, and nuts will markedly blunt the post-meal increase in glucose, triglycerides, and inflammation. Additionally, lean protein, vinegar, fish oil, tea, cinnamon, calorie restriction, weight loss, exercise, and low-dose to moderate-dose alcohol each positively impact post-prandial dysmetabolism.** Experimental and epidemiological studies indicate that eating patterns, such as the traditional Mediterranean or Okinawan diets, that incorporate these types of foods and beverages reduce inflammation and cardiovascular risk. This anti-inflammatory diet should be considered for the primary and secondary prevention of coronary artery disease and diabetes.

Seaweed and Weight Loss

It seems one weight loss strategy used across Asia comes from the sea. Quite amazingly, seaweed can block up to seventy five percent of the fat in the meal you are eating.

Source: Obes Rev. 2013 Feb;14(2):129-44. Epub 2012 Nov 12.
Title: Review: efficacy of alginate supplementation in relation to appetite regulation and metabolic risk factors: evidence from animal and human studies.

Authors: Georg Jensen M1, Pedersen C, Kristensen M, Frost G, Astrup A.

Abstract: This review provides a critical update on human and animal studies investigating the effect of alginate supplementation on appetite regulation, glycaemic and insulinemic responses, and lipid metabolism with discussion of the evidence on potential mechanisms, efficacy and tolerability. Dependent on vehicle applied for alginate supplementation, the majority of animal and human studies suggest that alginate consumption does suppress satiety and to some extent energy intake. **Only one long-term intervention trial found effects on weight loss. In addition, alginates seem to exhibit beneficial influence on postprandial glucose absorption and insulin response in animals and humans.** However, alginate supplementation was only found to have cholesterol-lowering properties in animals. Several mechanisms have been suggested for the positive effect observed, which involve delayed gastric emptying, increased viscosity of digesta and slowed nutrient absorption in the small intestine upon alginate gel formation. Despite reasonable efficacy and tolerability from the acute or short-term studies, we still realize there is a critical need for development of optimal alginate types and vehicles as well as studies on further long-term investigation on alginate supplementation in humans before inferring that it could be useful in the management of obesity and the metabolic syndrome.

Turmeric, Onions, Garlic

Certain flavors are good for the health, including the indian spice turmeric and the universal flavors of onion and garlic.

FREE FULLTEXT
Source: Asia Pac J Clin Nutr. 2008;17 Suppl 1:265-8.
Title: Traditional Indian spices and their health significance.
Author: Krishnaswamy K.
Abstract: India has been recognized all over the world for spices and medicinal plants. Both exhibit a wide range of physiological and pharmacological properties. Current biomedical efforts are focused on their scientific merits, to provide science-based evidence for the traditional uses and to develop either functional foods or nutraceuticals. The Indian traditional medical systems use turmeric for wound healing, rheumatic disorders, gastrointestinal symptoms, deworming, rhinitis and as a cosmetic. Studies in India have explored its anti-inflammatory, cholekinetic and anti-oxidant potentials with the recent investigations focusing on its preventive effect on precarcinogenic, anti-inflammatory and anti atherosclerotic effects in biological systems both under in vitro and in vivo

conditions in animals and humans. **Both turmeric and curcumin were found to increase detoxifying enzymes, prevent DNA damage, improve DNA repair, decrease mutations and tumour formation and exhibit antioxidative potential in animals. Limited clinical studies suggest that turmeric can significantly impact excretion of mutagens in urine in smokers and regress precancerous palatal lesions. It reduces DNA adducts and micronuclei in oral epithelial cells. It prevents formation of nitroso compounds both in vivo and in vitro. It delays induced cataract in diabetes and reduces hyperlipidemia in obese rats.** Recently several molecular targets have been identified for therapeutic / preventive effects of turmeric. Fenugreek seeds, a rich source of soluble fiber used in Indian cuisine reduces blood glucose and lipids and can be used as a food adjuvant in diabetes. Similarly garlic, onions, and ginger have been found to modulate favourably the process of carcinogenesis.

Calcium Helps

FREE FULLTEXT
Source: PLoS One. 2014 Oct 15;9(10):e108094. doi: 10.1371/journal.pone.0108094. eCollection 2014.
Title: Calcium supplementation increases blood creatinine concentration in a randomized controlled trial.
Authors: Barry EL1, Mott LA1, Melamed ML2, Rees JR1, Ivanova A3, Sandler RS4, Ahnen DJ5, Bresalier

RS6,Summers RW7, Bostick RM8, Baron JA9.

Abstract: BACKGROUND:: Calcium supplements are widely used among older adults for osteoporosis prevention and treatment. However, their effect on creatinine levels and kidney function has not been well studied.

METHODS: We investigated the effect of calcium supplementation on blood creatinine concentration in a randomized controlled trial of colorectal adenoma chemoprevention conducted between 2004-2013 at 11 clinical centers in the United States. Healthy participants (N=1,675) aged 45-75 with a history of colorectal adenoma were assigned to daily supplementation with calcium (1200 mg, as carbonate), vitamin D3 (1000 IU), both, or placebo for three or five years. Changes in blood creatinine and total calcium concentration were measured after one year of treatment and multiple linear regression was used to estimate effects on creatinine concentrations.

RESULTS: After one year of treatment, blood creatinine was 0.013 ± 0.006 mg/dL higher on average among participants randomized to calcium compared to placebo after adjustment for other determinants of creatinine (P=0.03). However, the effect of calcium treatment appeared to be larger among participants who consumed the most alcohol (2-6 drinks/day) or whose estimated glomerular filtration rate (eGFR) was less than 60 ml/min/1.73 m2 at baseline. The effect of calcium treatment on creatinine was only partially mediated by a concomitant increase in blood total calcium concentration and was independent of randomized vitamin D treatment. There did not appear to be further increases in creatinine after the first year of calcium treatment.

CONCLUSIONS: **Among healthy adults participating in a randomized clinical trial, daily supple-**

mentation with 1200 mg of elemental calcium caused a small increase in blood creatinine. If confirmed, this finding may have implications for clinical and public health recommendations for calcium supplementation.

Components of the Traditional Latin American Healthy Diet

Beans and Health

In Latin America and the East they use more beans in their cuisines than the United States. Maybe that is one reason they have been historically slimmer than people in the United States?

Source: J Med Food. 2013 Mar;16(3):185-98. doi: 10.1089/jmf.2011.0238. Epub 2013 Feb 11.
Title: Nutritional quality of legumes, and their role in cardiometabolic risk prevention: a review.
Authors: Bouchenak M, Lamri-Senhadji M.
Abstract: Legumes (including alfalfa, clover, lupins, green beans and peas, peanuts, soybeans, dry beans, broad beans, dry peas, chickpeas, and lentils) represent an important component of the human diet in several areas of the world, especially in the developing countries, where they complement the lack of proteins from cereals, roots, and tubers. In some regions of the world, legume seeds are the only protein supply in the diet. The health benefits of legume consumption have received rising interest from researchers, and their consumption and production extends worldwide. Among European countries,

higher legume consumption is observed around the Mediterranean, with per capita daily consumption between 8 and 23 g, while in Northern Europe, the daily consumption is less than 5 g per capita. The physiological effects of different legumes vary significantly. These differences may result from the polysaccharides composition, in particular, the quantity and variety of dietary fibers and starch, protein make-up, and variability in phytochemical content. The majority of legumes contain phytochemicals: bioactive compounds, including enzyme inhibitors, phytohemagglutinins (lectins), phytoestrogens, oligosaccharides, saponins, and phenolic compounds, which play metabolic roles in humans who frequently consume these foods. Dietary intake of phytochemicals may provide health benefits, protecting against numerous diseases or disorders, such as coronary heart disease, diabetes, high blood pressure and inflammation. The synergistic or antagonistic effects of these phytochemical mixtures from food legumes, their interaction with other components of the diet, and the mechanism of their action have remained a challenge with regard to understanding the role of phytochemicals in health and diseases. **Their mitigating effects and the mechanism of their action need to be further addressed if we are to understand the role of phytochemicals in health and diseases. This review provides an overview of the nutritional quality of legumes and their potential contribution in cardiometabolic risk prevention.**

Avocados- good for the heart and Nervous System

An excuse to eat guacamole? Is that even necessary?

<u>FREE FULLTEXT</u>
Source: Crit Rev Food Sci Nutr. 2013;53(7):738-50.
doi: 10.1080/10408398.2011.556759.
Title: Hass avocado composition and potential
health effects.

Authors: Dreher ML, Davenport AJ.

Abstract: Hass avocados, the most common commercial avocado cultivars in the world, contain a variety of essential nutrients and important phytochemicals. Although the official avocado serving is one-fifth of a fruit (30 g), according to NHANES analysis the average consumption is one-half an avocado (68 g), which provides a nutrient and phytochemical dense food consisting of the following: dietary fiber (4.6 g), total sugar (0.2 g), potassium (345 mg), sodium (5.5 mg), magnesium (19.5 mg), vitamin A (43 µg), vitamin C (6.0 mg), vitamin E (1.3 mg), vitamin K1 (14 µg), folate (60 mg), vitamin B-6 (0.2 mg), niacin (1.3 mg), pantothenic acid (1.0 mg), riboflavin (0.1 mg), choline (10 mg), lutein/zeaxanthin (185 µg), phytosterols (57 mg), and high-monounsaturated fatty acids (6.7 g) and 114 kcals or 1.7 kcal/g. The avocado oil consists of 71% monounsaturated fatty acids (MUFA), 13% polyunsaturated fatty acids (PUFA), and 16% saturated fatty acids (SFA), which helps to promote healthy blood lipid profiles and enhance the bioavailability of fat soluble vitamins and phytochemicals from the avocado or other fruits and vegetables, naturally low in fat, which are consumed with avocados. **There are eight preliminary clinical studies showing that avocado consumption helps support cardiovascular health. Exploratory studies** suggest that avocados may support weight management and healthy aging.

Chocolate and Heart Health

You are kidding? Chocolate is good for the heart? Yes. In moderation, dark chocolate is also good for weight loss due to the speeding up of the mitochondria in the cells due to catechins.

Source: Vascul Pharmacol. 2015 May 27. pii: S1537-1891(15)00113-5. doi: 10.1016/j.vph.2015.05.011.
Title: The cardiovascular benefits of dark chocolate.
Authors: Kerimi A, Williamson G2.
Abstract: Dark chocolate contains many biologically active components, such as catechins, procyanidins and theobromine from cocoa, together with added sucrose and lipids. All of these can directly or indirectly affect the cardiovascular system by multiple mechanisms. **Intervention studies on healthy and metabolically-dysfunctional volunteers have suggested that cocoa improves blood pressure, platelet aggregation and endothelial function.** The effect of chocolate is more convoluted since the sucrose and lipid may transiently and negatively impact on endothelial function, partly through insulin signalling and nitric oxide bioavailability. However, few studies have attempted to dissect out the role of the individual components and have not explored their possible interactions. For intervention studies, the situation is complex since suitable placebos are often not available, and some benefits may only be observed in individuals showing mild metabolic
82

dysfunction. For chocolate, the effects of some of the components, such as sugar and epicatechin on FMD, may oppose each other, or alternatively in some cases may act together, such as theobromine and epicatechin. Although clearly cocoa provides some cardiovascular benefits according to many human intervention studies, the exact components, their interactions and molecular mechanisms are still under debate.

Components of the European Healthy Diet

Red Wine, Resveratrol and Apigenin

Red wine is very anti-inflammatory and, in part, resveratrol, is the reason the French can eat a high-fat diet and remain so heart-healthy. Apigenin and resveratrol are synergistic.

Source: Cell Mol Life Sci. 2015 Apr;72(8):1473-88. doi: 10.1007/s00018-014-1808-8. Epub 2014 Dec 30.
Title: *Metabolic effects of resveratrol: addressing the controversies.*
Authors: Bitterman JL, Chung JH.
Abstract: Resveratrol, a polyphenol found in a number of plant-based foods such as red wine, has received a great deal of attention for its diverse array of healthful effects. **Beneficial effects of resveratrol are diverse; they include improvement of mitochondrial function, protection against obesity and obesity-related diseases such as type-2 diabetes, suppression of inflammation and cancer**

cell growth and protection against cardiovascular dysfunction, just to name a few. Investigations into the metabolic effects of resveratrol are furthest along and now include a number of clinical trials, which have yielded mixed results. There are a number of controversies surrounding resveratrol that have not been resolved. Here, we will review these controversies with particular emphasis on its mechanism of metabolic action and how lessons from resveratrol may help develop therapies that harness the effects of resveratrol but without the undesirable properties of resveratrol.

Polyphenols

Keep drinking that coffee! It's great for your liver and your heart! Coffee is the number one source of antioxidants in the American diet.

FREE FULLTEXT
Source: Curr Atheroscler Rep. 2013 May;15(5):324. doi: 10.1007/s11883-013-0324-x.
Title: Polyphenols, inflammation, and cardiovascular disease.
Authors: Tangney CC, Rasmussen HE.
Abstract: **Polyphenols are compounds found in foods such as tea, coffee, cocoa, olive oil, and red wine and have been studied to determine if their intake may modify cardiovascular disease (CVD) risk. Historically, biologic actions of polyphenols have been attributed to antioxidant activities, but recent evidence suggests that immunomodulatory and vasodilatory properties of polyphenols**

may also contribute to CVD risk reduction. These properties will be discussed, and recent epidemiological evidence and intervention trials will be reviewed. Further identification of polyphenols in foods and accurate assessment of exposures through measurement of biomarkers (i.e., polyphenol metabolites) could provide the needed impetus to examine the impact of polyphenol-rich foods on CVD intermediate outcomes (especially those signifying chronic inflammation) and hard endpoints among high risk patients. Although we have mechanistic insight into how polyphenols may function in CVD risk reduction, further research is needed before definitive recommendations for consumption can be made.

Components of A Healthy Diet from Africa and the Middle East

Coffee

J Am Coll Cardiol. 2013 Sep 17;62(12):1043-51. doi: 10.1016/j.jacc.2013.06.035. Epub 2013 Jul 17.
Effects of habitual coffee consumption on cardiometabolic disease, cardiovascular health, and all-cause mortality.

O'Keefe JH1, Bhatti SK, Patil HR, DiNicolantonio JJ, Lucan SC, Lavie CJ.

Abstract: Coffee, after water, is the most widely consumed beverage in the United States, and is the principal source of caffeine intake among adults.

The biological effects of coffee may be substantial and are not limited to the actions of caffeine. Coffee is a complex beverage containing hundreds of biologically active compounds, and the health effects of chronic coffee intake are wide ranging. From a cardiovascular (CV) standpoint, coffee consumption may reduce the risk of type 2 diabetes mellitus and hypertension, as well as other conditions associated with CV risk such as obesity and depression; but it may adversely affect lipid profiles depending on how the beverage is prepared. Regardless, **a growing body of data suggests that habitual coffee consumption is neutral to beneficial regarding the risks of a variety of adverse CV outcomes including coronary heart disease, congestive heart failure, arrhythmias, and stroke. Moreover, large epidemiological studies suggest that regular coffee drinkers have reduced risks of mortality, both CV and all-cause. The potential benefits also include protection against neurodegenerative diseases, improved asthma control, and lower risk of select gastrointestinal diseases.** A daily intake of 2 to 3 cups of coffee appears to be safe and is associated with neutral to beneficial effects for most of the studied health outcomes. However, most of the data on coffee's health effects are based on observational data, with very few randomized, controlled studies, and association does not prove causation. Additionally, the possible advantages of regular coffee consumption have to be weighed against potential risks (which are mostly related to its high caffeine content) including anxiety, insomnia, tremulousness, and palpitations, as well as bone loss and possibly increased risk of fractures.

African Mango?

There are conflicting studies on African Mango, it may help weight loss as the following study purports, or it may not.

FREE FULLTEXT
Source Holist Nurs Pract. 2011 Jul-Aug;25(4):215-7.
doi: 10.1097/HNP.0b013e318222735a.
Title: African mango (IGOB131): a proprietary seed extract of Irvingia gabonensis is found to be effective in reducing body weight and improving metabolic parameters in overweight humans.
Author: Ross SM1.

Black Seed and Health

FREE FULLTEXT
Source: Evid Based Complement Alternat Med. 2014;2014:724658. doi: 10.1155/2014/724658. Epub 2014 May 18.
Title: Therapeutic Implications of Black Seed and Its Constituent Thymoquinone in the Prevention of Cancer through Inactivation and Activation of Molecular Pathways.
Authors: Rahmani AH1, Alzohairy MA1, Khan MA2, Aly SM3.

Abstract: The cancer is probably the most dreaded disease in both men and women and also major health problem worldwide. Despite its high prevalence, the exact molecular mechanisms of the development and progression are not fully understood. The current chemotherapy/radiotherapy regime used to treat cancer shows adverse side effect and may alter gene functions. Natural products are generally safe, effective, and less expensive substitutes of anti-cancer chemotherapeutics. Based on previous studies of their potential therapeutic uses, Nigella sativa and its constituents may be proved as good therapeutic options in the prevention of cancer. Black seeds are used as staple food in the Middle Eastern Countries for thousands of years and also in the treatment of diseases. Earlier studies have shown that N. sativa and its constituent thymoquinone (TQ) have important roles in the prevention and treatment of cancer by modulating cell signaling pathways. In this review, we summarize the role of N. sativa and its constituents TQ in the prevention of cancer through the activation or inactivation of molecular cell signaling pathways.

The Role of Fruit, Veggies, and Fermentation in Weight Loss and Natural Diabetes Control

The Meaning of Fruit and Vegetable Colors

FREE FULLTEXT
Source: J Nutr. 2001 Nov;131(11 Suppl):3078S-81S.
Title: Applying science to changing dietary patterns.
Authors: Heber D, Bowerman S.
Abstract: The intake of 400-600 g/d of fruits and vegetables is associated with reduced incidence of many common forms of cancer. These foods contain phytochemicals that can modulate gene expression to

inhibit carcinogenesis via multiple pathways. Many phytochemicals are colorful, providing an easy way to communicate increased diversity of fruits and vegetables to the public. Red foods contain lycopene, the pigment in tomatoes, which is localized in the prostate gland and may be involved in maintaining prostate health. Yellow-green vegetables, such as corn and leafy greens, contain lutein and zeaxanthin, which are localized in the retina where age-related macular degeneration occurs. Red-purple foods contain anthocyanins, which are powerful antioxidants found in red apples, grapes, berries and wine. Orange foods, including carrots, mangos, apricots, pumpkin and winter squash, contain beta-carotene. Orange-yellow foods, including oranges, tangerines and lemons contain citrus flavonoids. Green foods, including broccoli, Brussels sprouts and kale, contain glucosinolates. White-green foods in the onion family contain allyl sulfides. Consumers are advised to ingest one serving of each of the above groups daily, putting this recommendation within the National Cancer Institute and American Institute for Cancer Research guidelines of five to nine servings per day. The color code provides simplification, but it is also important as a way to help consumers to find common fruits and vegetables easily while traveling, eating in restaurants or working. At home, simple ways of preparing foods rapidly and easily are needed to influence dietary patterns.

Citrus and Weight Loss

FREE FULLTEXT
Source: Adv Nutr. 2014 Jul 14;5(4):404-17. doi: 10.3945/an.113.005603. Print 2014 Jul.
Title; Effect of citrus flavonoids, naringin and naringenin, on metabolic syndrome and their mechanisms of action.
Authors: Alam MA, Subhan N, Rahman MM, Uddin SJ, Reza HM, Sarker SD.
Abstract: Flavonoids are important natural compounds with diverse biologic activities. Citrus flavonoids constitute an important series of flavonoids. Naringin and its aglycone naringenin belong to this series of flavonoids and were found to display strong anti-inflammatory and antioxidant activities. **Several lines of investigation suggest that naringin supplementation is beneficial for the treatment of obesity, diabetes, hypertension, and metabolic syndrome.** A number of molecular mechanisms underlying its beneficial activities have been elucidated. However, their effect on obesity and metabolic disorder remains to be fully established. Moreover, the therapeutic uses of these flavonoids are significantly limited by the lack of adequate clinical evidence. This review aims to explore the biologic activities of these compounds, particularly on lipid metabolism in obesity, oxidative stress, and inflammation in context of metabolic syndrome.

Grapefruit and Weight Loss

FREE FULLTEXT
Source: Nutr Metab (Lond). 2011 Feb 2;8(1):8. doi: 10.1186/1743-7075-8-8.
Title: Effects of grapefruit, grapefruit juice and water preloads on energy balance, weight loss, body composition, and cardiometabolic risk in free-living obese adults.
Authors: Silver HJ, Dietrich MS, Niswender KD.
Abstract: BACKGROUND: Reducing dietary energy density has proven to be an effective strategy to reduce energy intakes and promote weight control. This effect appears most robust when a low energy dense preload is consumed before meals. Yet, much discussion continues regarding the optimal form of a preload. The purpose of the present study was to compare effects of a solid (grapefruit), liquid (grapefruit juice) and water preload consumed prior to breakfast, lunch and dinner in the context of caloric restriction. METHODS: Eighty-five obese adults (BMI 30-39.9) were randomly assigned to (127 g) grapefruit (GF), grapefruit juice (GFJ) or water preload for 12 weeks after completing a 2-week caloric restriction phase. Preloads were matched for weight, calories, water content, and energy density. Weekly measures included blood pressure, weight, anthropometry and 24-hour dietary intakes. Resting energy expenditure, body composition, physical performance and cardiometabolic risk biomarkers were assessed.
RESULTS: The total amount (grams) of food consumed did not change over time. Yet, after preloads were combined with caloric restriction, average dietary energy density and total energy intakes decreased by 20-29% from baseline values. **Subjects**

experienced 7.1% weight loss overall, with significant decreases in percentage body, trunk, android and gynoid fat, as well as waist circumferences (-4.5 cm). However, differences were not statistically significant among groups. Nevertheless, the amount and direction of change in serum HDL-cholesterol levels in GF (+6.2%) and GFJ (+8.2%) preload groups was significantly greater than water preload group (-3.7%).

CONCLUSIONS: These data indicate that incorporating consumption of a low energy dense dietary preload in a caloric restricted diet is a highly effective weight loss strategy. But, the form of the preload did not have differential effects on energy balance, weight loss or body composition. It is notable that subjects in GF and GFJ preload groups experienced significantly greater benefits in lipid profiles.

Kale, Cabbage, Collard Greens, Brussel Sprouts: the Brassica Vegetables

Cabbage used to be called "The poor man's medicine", for good reason. Sometimes peasant food is pleasant food and great for the health.

FREE FULLTEXT
Source: Rocz Panstw Zakl Hig. 2012;63(4):389-95.
Title: The beneficial effects of Brassica vegetables on human health.
Authors: Kapusta-Duch J, Kopeć A, Piatkowska E, Borczak B, Leszczyńska T.

Abstract: The products of plant origin are a rich source of biologically active substances, both nutritive and referred as anti-nutritive. A large group of these compounds are substances with antioxidant activity that fights against free radicals. In the family of Brassicaceae vegetables, Brassica, is the largest and most widely consumed a group of plants in Europe and all over the world. They are characterized by different levels of nutrients. However because of their large and frequent consumption, they may become a significant source of nutrients and bioactive compounds in the daily diet. **The beneficial effects of Brassica vegetables on human health have been somewhat linked to phytochemicals. They prevent oxidative stress, induce detoxification enzymes, stimulate immune system, decrease the risk of cancers, inhibit malignant transformation and carcinogenic mutations, as well as, reduce proliferation of cancer cells.** Brassica vegetables contain a lot of valuable metabolites, which are effective in chemoprevention of cancer, what has been already documented by numerous studies. Due to the presence of vitamins C and E, carotenoids and antioxidant enzymes such as catalase, superoxide dismutase (SOD) and peroxidase, these vegetables are considerable source of antioxidants, and due to the presence of polyphenols and the sulfur-organic compounds exert also antimutagenic action. Moreover, these vegetables are also rich in glucosinolates, which are unstable compounds and undergo degradation into biologically active indoles and isothiocyanates under the influence of enzyme presented in plant tissues-myrosynase. These substances through the induction of enzymatic systems I and II phase of xenobiotics metabolism may affect the elimination or neutralization of carcinogenic and mutagenic factors, and consequently inhibit DNA methylation and cancer development. Despite many healthy benefits upon eating of cruciferous vegetables, it has been also seen a negative impact of their certain ingredients on the human body.

Apples and Weight Loss

The old saying seems true that an apple a day keeps the doctor away. Apple peels contain Ursolic acid which is present in many fruits and herbs used in daily life e.g. basil,bilberries, cranberries, elder flower, peppermint, rosemary, lavender,oregano, thyme, hawthorn, and prunes. Ursolic acid grows reserves of the fat burning type of fat, brown fat, along with exercise, and melatonin rich foods such as almonds, tomatoes, tart cherries, cardamom, and coriander.

FREE FULLTEXT

Source: Nutrients. 2015 May 26;7(6):3959-3998.
Title: Apples and Cardiovascular Health-Is the Gut Microbiota a Core Consideration?
Authors: Koutsos A, Tuohy KM, Lovegrove JA.
Abstract: **There is now considerable scientific evidence that a diet rich in fruits and vegetables can improve human health and protect against chronic diseases.** However, it is not clear whether different fruits and vegetables have distinct beneficial effects. Apples are among the most frequently consumed fruits and a rich source of polyphenols and fiber. A major proportion of the bioactive compo-

nents in apples, including the high molecular weight polyphenols, escape absorption in the upper gastro-intestinal tract and reach the large intestine relatively intact. There, they can be converted by the colonic microbiota to bioavailable and biologically active compounds with systemic effects, in addition to modulating microbial composition. Epidemiological studies have identified associations between frequent apple consumption and reduced risk of chronic diseases such as cardiovascular disease. Human and animal intervention studies demonstrate beneficial effects on lipid metabolism, vascular function and inflammation but only a few studies have attempted to link these mechanistically with the gut microbiota. This review will focus on the reciprocal interaction between apple components and the gut microbiota, the potential link to cardiovascular health and the possible mechanisms of action.

Fermented Fruits and Vegetables and Health
They taste good, and they're good for you!

FREE FULLTEXT
Source: Biotechnol Res Int. 2014;2014:250424. doi: 10.1155/2014/250424. Epub 2014 May 28.
Title: Fermented fruits and vegetables of Asia: a potential source of probiotics.
Authors: Swain MR, Anandharaj M, Ray RC, Parveen Rani R.
Abstract: As world population increases, lactic acid fermentation is expected to become an important role in preserving fresh vegetables, fruits, and other

food items for feeding humanity in developing countries. However, several fermented fruits and vegetables products (Sauerkraut, Kimchi, Gundruk, Khalpi, Sinki, etc.) have a long history in human nutrition from ancient ages and are associated with the several social aspects of different communities. Among the food items, fruits and vegetables are easily perishable commodities due to their high water activity and nutritive values. These conditions are more critical in tropical and subtropical countries which favour the growth of spoilage causing microorganisms. Lactic acid fermentation increases shelf life of fruits and vegetables and also enhances several beneficial properties, including nutritive value and flavours, and reduces toxicity. Fermented fruits and vegetables can be used as a potential source of probiotics as they harbour several lactic acid bacteria such as Lactobacillus plantarum, L. pentosus, L. brevis, L. acidophilus, L. fermentum, Leuconostoc fallax, and L. mesenteroides. As a whole, the traditionally fermented fruits and vegetables not only serve as food supplements but also attribute towards health benefits. This review aims to describe some important Asian fermented fruits and vegetables and their significance as a potential source of probiotics.

Yogurt and Kefir do a Body Good
Not all yogurt is good for you. Maybe try an organic yoghurt that is not sweetened. That way you cut out the excess sugar.

FREE FULLTEXT
Source: Am J Clin Nutr. 2014 May;99(5
Suppl):1209S-11S. doi: 10.3945/ajcn.113.073429.
Epub 2014 Mar 19.
Title: Introduction to the yogurt in nutrition initiative and the First Global Summit on the health effects of yogurt.

Authors: Donovan SM1, Shamir R.

Abstract: Yogurt has been part of the human diet for thousands of years, and during that time a number of health benefits have been associated with its consumption. The goal of the First Global Summit on the Health Effects of Yogurt was to review and evaluate the strength of current scientific knowledge with regard to the health benefits of yogurt and to identify areas where further research is needed. **The evidence base for the benefits of yogurt in promoting bone health, maintaining health throughout the life cycle, improving diet quality, and reducing the incidence of chronic diseases, such as obesity, metabolic syndrome, and cardiovascular disease, was presented.** When assessing a complex food matrix, rather than specific nutrients, scientists and consumers are faced with new challenges as to how a food item's quality or necessity would be judged as part of an individual's whole diet. To tackle this challenge, speakers described methods for assessing the nutrient density of foods and its application to yogurt, use of yogurt for lactose intolerance, and the cost-effectiveness of yogurt and dairy products in reducing health care expenses. Last, speakers described the role of dairy products in global public health and nutrition, the scientific basis for current dairy recommendations, and future scientific and policy needs related to dairy and yogurt recommendations.

Berries Protect against Diabetes

The polyphenols in berries are good for you, period. Think back to the times of the hunter-gatherers. They knew how to eat.

Source: Biofactors. 2005;23(4):189-95.
Title: The inhibitory effects of berry polyphenols on digestive enzymes.
Authors: McDougall GJ, Stewart D.
Abstract: The evidence for the effect of polyphenol components of berries on digestive enzymes is reviewed. Anthocyanins inhibit alpha-glucosidase activity and can reduce blood glucose levels after starch-rich meals, a proven clinical therapy for controlling type II diabetes. Ellagitannins inhibit alpha-amylase activity and there is potential for synergistic effects on starch degradation after ingestion of berries such as raspberries and strawberries, which contain substantial amounts of ellagitannins and anthocyanins. A range of berry polyphenols (e.g. flavonols, anthocyanidins, ellagitannins and proanthocyanidins) can inhibit protease activities at levels which could affect protein digestion in the gastrointestinal tract. In contrast, potential for the inhibition of gastrointestinal lipase activity, a proven therapeutic target for the control of obesity through reduced fat digestion, may be limited to proanthocyanidins. Taking into account the manifold possible synergies for inhibition of starch, protein and/or lipid digestion by the spectrum of polyphenol components present within berry species, the inhibition of digestive enzymes by dietary polyphenols may represent an under-reported mechanism for delivering some of the health benefits attributed to a diet rich in fruit and vegetables.

Vinegar and Weight Loss

Source: J Am Coll Nutr. 2005 Jun;24(3):158-65.
Title: Strategies for healthy weight loss: from vitamin C to the glycemic response.
Author: Johnston CS.

Abstract: America is experiencing a major obesity epidemic. The ramifications of this epidemic are immense since obesity is associated with chronic metabolic abnormalities such as insulin resistance, dyslipidemia, and heart disease. Reduced physical activity and/or increased energy intakes are important factors in this epidemic. Additionally, a genetic susceptibility to obesity is associated with gene polymorphisms affecting biochemical pathways that regulate fat oxidation, energy expenditure, or energy intake. However, these pathways are also impacted by specific foods and nutrients. Vitamin C status is inversely related to body mass. Individuals with adequate vitamin C status oxidize 30% more fat during a moderate exercise bout than individuals with low vitamin C status; thus, vitamin C depleted individuals may be more resistant to fat mass loss. Food choices can impact post-meal satiety and hunger. High-protein foods promote postprandial thermogenesis and greater satiety as compared to high-carbohydrate, low-fat foods; thus, diet regimens high in protein foods may improve diet compliance and diet effectiveness. **Vinegar and peanut ingestion can reduce the glycemic effect of a meal, a phenomenon that has been related to satiety and reduced food consumption.** Thus, the effectiveness of regular exercise and a prudent diet for weight loss may be enhanced by attention to specific diet details.

Nutraceuticals

CoQ10

Long term, CoQ10 may prevent nerve damage in diabetes, and it can also be of some help in weight loss and the production of energy.

Source: Neurobiol Dis. 2013 Oct;58:169-78. doi: 10.1016/j.nbd.2013.05.003. Epub 2013 May 16.
Title: Diabetic neuropathic pain development in type 2 diabetic mouse model and the prophylactic and therapeutic effects of coenzyme Q10.
Authors: Zhang YP, Song CY, Yuan Y, Eber A, Rodriguez Y, Levitt RC, Takacs P, Yang Z, Goldberg R, Candiotti KA.

Abstract: ...CONCLUSION: This model may be useful in understanding the mechanisms of neuropathic pain in type 2 DM induced neuropathic pain and may facilitate preclinical testing of therapies. **CoQ10 may decrease oxidative stress in the central and peripheral nervous system by acting as an anti-oxidant and free-radical scavenger. These results suggest that CoQ10 might be a reasonable preventative strategy for long-term use and using CoQ10 treatment may be a safe and effective long-term approach in the treatment of diabetic neuropathy.**
Vitamin D

FREE FULLTEXT
Source: Perm J. 2014 Fall;18(4):32-9. doi: 10.7812/TPP/14-016.
Title: Prevalence of hypovitaminosis D and its association with comorbidities of childhood obesity.

Authors: Williams R, Novick M, Lehman E.
Abstract: PURPOSE: Our study sought to further delineate the prevalence of hypovitaminosis D and its relationship to comorbidities of childhood obesity. METHODS: We conducted a retrospective chart review from 155 obese children aged 5 to 19 years who attended the Penn State Children's Hospital Pediatric Multidisciplinary Weight Loss Program from November 2009 through November 2010. We determined the incidence of hypovitaminosis D and examined its association with comorbidities including elevated blood pressure, diabetes, acanthosis nigricans, depression, hyperlipidemia, hyperinsulinemia, and abnormal liver function test results, as well as age, sex, and geographic location. RESULTS: Under the latest Institute of Medicine definitions, vitamin D deficiency (< 20 ng/mL) and insufficiency (20-29 ng/mL) was present in 40% and 38% of children, respectively. The prevalence of vitamin D deficiency was 27.8% in children aged 5 to 9 years, 35.4% in children aged 10 to 14 years, and 50.9% of children aged 15 years or older. Older age, African-American race, winter/spring season, higher insulin level, total number of comorbidities, and polycystic ovary syndrome (in girls) were significantly associated with vitamin D deficiency. African-American race, winter/spring season, hyperinsulinemia, elevated systolic blood pressure, urban location, and total numbers of comorbidities were significantly associated with hypovitaminosis D (< 30 ng/mL). CONCLUSIONS: **Hypovitaminosis D is associated with several medical comorbidities in obese children. Given the large percentage of children, even in our youngest age group, who are vitamin D deficient, obese children should be considered for routine vitamin D screening.**

Vitamin E

Fat soluble vitamin E is even more important for those with fatty-liver disease.

FREE FULLTEXT
Source: Niger J Clin Pract. 2015 Nov-Dec;18(6):703-12. doi: 10.4103/1119-3077.163288.
Title: Nonalcoholic fatty liver disease: Synopsis of current developments.
Authors: Onyekwere CA, Ogbera AO, Samaila AA, Balogun BO, Abdulkareem FB.

Abstract: Non-alcoholic fatty liver disease (NAFLD) which is defined as the accumulation of fat>5% of liver weight is increasingly becoming an important cause of chronic liver disease. This article tries to chronicle advances that have occurred in the understanding of the pathogenesis, pathology as well as the management of this disease. We have done a Medline search on published work on the subject and reviewed major conference proceedings in the preceding years. The Pathogenesis involves a multi-hit process in which increased accumulation of triglycerides in face of insulin resistance results in increased susceptibility to inflammatory damage mediated by increased expression of inflammatory cytokines and adipokines, oxidative stress and mitochondrial dysfunction, endoplasmic reticulum stress and gut derived endotoxemia. An interplay of multiple metabolic genetic expression and environmental factors however determine which patient with NAFLD will progress from simple steatosis to non-alcoholic steatohepatitis (NASH) and liver cirrhosis. The minimum criteria for diagnosis of NASH are steatosis, ballooning and lobular inflammation;

fibrosis is not required. The NASH Clinical Research Network (CRN), histological scoring system is used to grade and stage the disease for standardization. The management of NAFLD consists of treating liver disease as well as associated metabolic co-morbidities such as obesity, hyperlipidaemia, insulin resistance and type 2 diabetes mellitus (T2DM). Patient education is important as their insight and commitment is pivotal, and lifestyle modification is the first line of treatment. Improvement in liver histology in non-diabetic NASH patients has been reported with use of Vitamin E. Other liver-related therapies under investigations include pentoxyfiylins, Caspar inhibitors, Resveratrol as well as probiotics. The prognosis (both overall and liver-related mortality) for simple steatosis is not different from that of the general population however.

Zinc

Take especial care not to overdo zinc. It can be very toxic.

FREE FULLTEXT
Source: Cell Mol Life Sci. 2013 Dec;70(23):4569-84. doi: 10.1007/s00018-013-1395-0. Epub 2013 Jun 13.
Title: Emerging roles of zinc finger proteins in regulating adipogenesis.
Authors: Wei S1, Zhang L, Zhou X, Du M, Jiang Z, Hausman GJ, Bergen WG, Zan L, Dodson MV.
Abstract: Proteins containing the zinc finger

domain(s) are named zinc finger proteins (ZFPs), one of the largest classes of transcription factors in eukaryotic genomes. A large number of ZFPs have been studied and many of them were found to be involved in regulating normal growth and development of cells and tissues through diverse signal transduction pathways. Recent studies revealed that a small but increasing number of ZFPs could function as key transcriptional regulators involved in adipogenesis. **Due to the prevalence of obesity and metabolic disorders, the investigation of molecular regulatory mechanisms of adipocyte development must be more completely understood in order to develop novel and long-term impact strategies for ameliorating obesity. In this review, we discuss recent work that has documented that ZFPs are important functional contributors to the regulation of adipogenesis.** Taken together, these data lead to the conclusion that ZFPs may become promising targets to combat human obesity.

Carnitine

Source: Clin Endocrinol (Oxf). 2015 Dec 15. doi: 10.1111/cen.13003. [Epub ahead of print]
Title: Oral carnitine supplementation reduces body weight and insulin resistance in women with polycystic ovary syndrome: a randomized, double-blind, placebo-controlled trial.
Authors: Samimi M, Jamilian M, Ebrahimi FA, Rahimi M, Tajbakhsh B, Asemi Z.
Abstract OBJECTIVE: Limited data are available evaluating the effects of oral carnitine supplementa-

tion on weight loss and metabolic profiles of women with polycystic ovary syndrome (PCOS). This study was designed to determine the effects of oral carnitine supplementation on weight loss, and glycaemic and lipid profiles in women with PCOS.

RESULTS: At the end of the 12 weeks, taking carnitine supplements resulted in a significant reduction in weight (-2.7±1.5 vs. +0.1±1.8 kg, P<0.001), BMI (-1.1±0.6 vs. +0.1±0.7 kg/m2 , P<0.001), waist circumference (WC) (-2.0±1.3 vs. -0.3±2.0 cm, P<0.001) and hip circumference (HC) (-2.5±1.5 vs. -0.3±1.8 cm, P<0.001) compared with placebo. In addition, compared with placebo, carnitine administration in women with PCOS led to a significant reduction in fasting plasma glucose (-0.38±0.36 vs. +0.11±0.97 mmol/L, P=0.01), serum insulin levels (-14.39±25.80 vs. +3.01±37.25 pmol/L, P=0.04), homeostasis model of assessment-insulin resistance (-0.61±1.03 vs. +0.11±1.43, P=0.04) and dehydroepiandrosterone sulfate (-3.64±7.00 vs. -0.59±3.20 µmol/L, P=0.03). CONCLUSIONS: **Overall, 12 weeks of carnitine administration in PCOS women resulted in reductions in weight, BMI, WC and HC, and beneficial effects on glycaemic control;** however, it did not affect lipid profiles or free testosterone.

Taurine

Source: Amino Acids. 2012 May;42(5):1529-39. doi: 10.1007/s00726-011-0883-5. Epub 2011 Mar 25.

Title: The potential usefulness of taurine on diabetes mellitus and its complications.

Authors: Ito T, Schaffer SW, Azuma J.

Abstract: Taurine (2-aminoethanesulfonic acid) is a free amino acid found ubiquitously in millimolar concentrations in all mammalian tissues. Taurine exerts a variety of biological actions, including antioxidation, modulation of ion movement, osmoregulation, modulation of neurotransmitters, and conjugation of bile acids, which may maintain physiological homeostasis. **Recently, data is accumulating that show the effectiveness of taurine against diabetes mellitus, insulin resistance and its complications, including retinopathy, nephropathy, neuropathy, atherosclerosis and cardiomyopathy, independent of hypoglycemic effect in several animal models.** The useful effects appear due to the multiple actions of taurine on cellular functions. This review summarizes the beneficial effects of taurine supplementation on diabetes mellitus and the molecular mechanisms underlying its effectiveness.

Turmeric

Source: Biofactors. 2013 Jan-Feb;39(1):78-87. doi: 10.1002/biof.1074. Epub 2013 Jan 22.
Title: Curcumin and obesity.

Author: Bradford PG

Abstract: Turmeric has been long recognized for its anti-inflammatory and health-promoting properties. Curcumin is one of the principal anti-inflammatory and healthful components of turmeric comprising

2-8% of most turmeric preparations. **Experimental evidence supports the activity of curcumin in promoting weight loss and reducing the incidence of obesity-related diseases.** With the discovery that obesity is characterized by chronic low-grade metabolic inflammation, phytochemicals like curcumin which have anti-inflammatory activity are being intensely investigated. Recent scientific research reveals that curcumin directly interacts with white adipose tissue to suppress chronic inflammation. In adipose tissue, curcumin inhibits macrophage infiltration and nuclear factor B (NF-B) activation induced by inflammatory agents. Curcumin reduces the expression of the potent proinflammatory adipokines tumor necrosis factor- (TNF), monocyte chemoattractant protein-1 (MCP-1), and plasminogen activator inhibitor type-1 (PAI-1), and it induces the expression of adiponectin, the principal anti-inflammatory agent secreted by adipocytes. Curcumin also has effects to inhibit adipocyte differentiation and to promote antioxidant activities. Through these diverse mechanisms curcumin reduces obesity and curtails the adverse health effects of obesity.

Foods to Minimize

Salt

FREE FULLTEXT
BMJ Open. 2013 Dec 23;3(12):e003733. doi: 10.1136/bmjopen-2013-003733.
Global, regional and national sodium intakes in 1990 and 2010: a systematic analysis of 24 h urinary

sodium excretion and dietary surveys worldwide. Powles J, Fahimi S, Micha R, Khatibzadeh S, Shi P, Ezzati M, Engell RE, Lim SS, Danaei G, Mozaffarian D; Global Burden of Diseases Nutrition and Chronic Diseases Expert Group (NutriCoDE). (127 more)

Abstract: OBJECTIVES: To estimate global, regional (21 regions) and national (187 countries) sodium intakes in adults in 1990 and 2010.

DESIGN: Bayesian hierarchical modelling using all identifiable primary sources.

DATA SOURCES AND ELIGIBILITY: We searched and obtained published and unpublished data from 142 surveys of 24 h urinary sodium and 103 of dietary sodium conducted between 1980 and 2010 across 66 countries. Dietary estimates were converted to urine equivalents based on 79 pairs of dual measurements.

MODELLING METHODS: Bayesian hierarchical modelling used survey data and their characteristics to estimate mean sodium intake, by sex, 5 years age group and associated uncertainty for persons aged 20+ in 187 countries in 1990 and 2010. Country-level covariates were national income/person and composition of food supplies.

MAIN OUTCOME MEASURES: Mean sodium intake (g/day) as estimable by 24 h urine collections, without adjustment for non-urinary losses.

RESULTS: In 2010, global mean sodium intake was 3.95 g/day (95% uncertainty interval: 3.89 to 4.01). This was nearly twice the WHO recommended limit of 2 g/day and equivalent to 10.06 (9.88-10.21) g/day of salt. Intake in men was 10% higher than in women; differences by age were small. Intakes were highest in East Asia, Central Asia and Eastern Europe (mean >4.2 g/day) and in Central Europe and

Middle East/North Africa (3.9-4.2 g/day). Regional mean intakes in North America, Western Europe and Australia/New Zealand ranged from 3.4 to 3.8 g/day. Intakes were lower (<3.3 g/day), but more uncertain, in sub-Saharan Africa and Latin America. Between 1990 and 2010, modest, but uncertain, increases in sodium intakes were identified.

CONCLUSIONS: **Sodium intakes exceed the recommended levels in almost all countries with small differences by age and sex. Virtually all populations would benefit from sodium reduction, supported by enhanced surveillance.**

Cochrane Database Syst Rev. 2003;(3):CD003656.
Reduced dietary salt for prevention of cardiovascular disease.

Hooper L1, Bartlett C, Davey Smith G, Ebrahim S.

Abstract: BACKGROUND: Restricting sodium intake in elevated blood pressure over short periods of time reduces blood pressure. Long term effects (on mortality, morbidity or blood pressure) of advice to reduce salt in patients with elevated or normal blood pressure are unclear.

OBJECTIVES: To assess in adults the long term effects (mortality, cardiovascular events, blood pressure, quality of life, weight, urinary sodium excretion, other nutrients and use of anti-hypertensive medications) of advice to restrict dietary sodium using all relevant randomised controlled trials.

SEARCH STRATEGY: The Cochrane Library, MEDLINE, EMBASE, bibliographies of included studies and related systematic reviews were searched for unconfounded randomised trials in healthy adults aiming to reduce sodium intake over at least 6 months. Attempts were made to trace unpublished or missed studies and authors of all included trials were contacted. There were no language restrictions. REVIEWER'S CONCLUSIONS: Intensive interventions, unsuited to primary care or population prevention programmes, provide only minimal reductions in blood pressure during long-term trials. Further evaluations to assess effects on morbidity and mortality outcomes are needed for populations as a whole and for patients with elevated blood pressure. Evidence from a large and small trial showed that a low sodium diet helps in maintenance of lower blood pressure following withdrawal of antihypertensives. If this is confirmed, with no increase in cardiovascular events, then targeting of comprehensive dietary and behavioural programmes in patients with elevated blood pressure requiring drug treatment would be justified.

Wheat and Anti-Nutrients

Wheat has anti-nutrients- Why is wheat so prevalent? There are much better sources of carbohydrates. I remember reading about the Pharaohs of Egypt, and how some suffered from diabetes. I thought to myself, what a modern condition for such an ancient ruler. The truth is that probably the Pharaohs were more or less sedentary and ate a lot of grain, including wheat, as opposed to the nuts and berries upon which our hunter-gatherer ancestors subsisted.

FREE FULLTEXT
Source: Nutrients. 2013 Mar 12;5(3):771-87. doi: 10.3390/nu5030771.

Title: *The dietary intake of wheat and other cereal grains and their role in inflammation.*
Authors: de Punder K, Pruimboom L.
Abstract: Wheat is one of the most consumed cereal grains worldwide and makes up a substantial part of the human diet. Although government-supported dietary guidelines in Europe and the U.S. advise individuals to eat adequate amounts of (whole) grain products per day, cereal grains contain "anti-nutrients," such as wheat gluten and wheat lectin, that in humans can elicit dysfunction and disease. In this review we discuss evidence from in vitro, in vivo and human intervention studies that describe how the consumption of wheat, but also other cereal grains, can contribute to the manifestation of chronic inflammation and autoimmune diseases by increasing intestinal permeability and initiating a pro-inflammatory immune response.

Trans Fats and Weight Gain

FREE FULLTEXT
Source: Postepy Hig Med Dosw (Online). 2010 Dec 27;64:650-8.
Title: [Dietary trans-fatty acids and metabolic syndrome].
Authors: Kochan Z, Karbowska J, Babicz-Zielińska E.
[Article in Polish]
Abstract: Trans-fatty acids (TFAs), products of partial hydrogenation of vegetable oils, have become more prevalent in our diet since the 1960s, when they re-

placed animal fats. TFAs also occur naturally in meat and dairy products from ruminants. There is growing evidence that dietary trans-fatty acids may increase the risk of metabolic syndrome. Several studies have demonstrated adverse effects of TFAs on plasma lipids and lipoproteins. In dietary trials, trans-fatty acids have been shown to raise the total cholesterol/HDL cholesterol ratio and Lp(a) levels in blood. Moreover, a high intake of TFAs has been associated with an increased risk of coronary heart disease. **Prospective cohort studies have shown that dietary trans-fatty acids promote abdominal obesity and weight gain. In addition, it appears that TFA consumption may be associated with the development of insulin resistance and type 2 diabetes.** The documented adverse health effects of TFAs emphasise the importance of efforts to reduce the content of partially hydrogenated vegetable oils in foods.

Eating Fast Food Causes Weight Gain

FREE FULLTEXT
Source: J Am Board Fam Med. 2008 Mar-Apr;21(2):135-40. doi: 10.3122/jabfm.2008.02.070034.
Title: Preventing or improving obesity by addressing specific eating patterns.
Authors: Greenwood JL, Stanford JB.
Abstract: The problem of obesity and overweight is an epidemic in the United States. Weight is a product of energy balance: energy intake versus energy expenditure. The purpose of this review is to identify

adult eating behaviors that are known to strongly affect the energy intake side of the energy balance and that may be readily amenable to prevention and intervention efforts in primary care. **Restaurant and fast food consumption, large portion sizes, and consumption of beverages with sugar added increase energy intake and are highly associated with weight gain and obesity.** Conversely, consumption of low energy dense food, ie, fruits and vegetables, and routine healthy breakfast consumption can help to maintain or lose weight. These distinct behaviors represent concrete negative and positive eating patterns on which primary care providers can focus when counseling overweight and obese patients. They also represent behavioral targets for designing and testing clinical interventions.

The Role of Exercise in Weight Loss and Diabetes Management

Strength Training and Basal Metabolism Rate (BMR)

FREE FULLTEXT
Source: J Clin Invest. 1990 Nov;86(5):1423-7.
Title: Skeletal muscle metabolism is a major determinant of resting energy expenditure.
Authors: Zurlo F, Larson K, Bogardus C, Ravussin E.
Abstract: Energy expenditure varies among people, independent of body size and composition, and persons with a "low" metabolic rate seem to be at higher

risk of gaining weight. To assess the importance of skeletal muscle metabolism as a determinant of metabolic rate, 24-h energy expenditure, basal metabolic rate (BMR), and sleeping metabolic rate (SMR) were measured by indirect calorimetry in 14 subjects (7 males, 7 females; 30 +/- 6 yr [mean +/- SD]; 79.1 +/- 17.3 kg; 22 +/- 7% body fat), and compared to forearm oxygen uptake. Values of energy expenditure were adjusted for individual differences in fat-free mass, fat mass, age, and sex. Adjusted BMR and SMR, expressed as deviations from predicted values, correlated with forearm resting oxygen uptake (ml O2/liter forearm) (r = 0.72, P less than 0.005 and r = 0.53, P = 0.05, respectively). **These findings suggest that differences in resting muscle metabolism account for part of the variance in metabolic rate among individuals and may play a role in the pathogenesis of obesity.**

Brown Fat and Basal Metabolism Rate

FREE FULLTEXT
Source: PLoS One. 2013 Oct 23;8(10):e77221. doi: 10.1371/journal.pone.0077221. eCollection 2013.
Title: Vagus nerve stimulation increases energy expenditure: relation to brown adipose tissue activity.
Authors: Vijgen GH, Bouvy ND, Leenen L, Rijkers K, Cornips E, Majoie M, Brans B, van Marken Lichtenbelt WD.
Abstract: BACKGROUND: Human brown adipose tissue (BAT) activity is inversely related to obesity

and positively related to energy expenditure. BAT is highly innervated and it is suggested the vagus nerve mediates peripheral signals to the central nervous system, there connecting to sympathetic nerves that innervate BAT. Vagus nerve stimulation (VNS) is used for refractory epilepsy, but is also reported to generate weight loss. We hypothesize VNS increases energy expenditure by activating BAT.

METHODS AND FINDINGS: Fifteen patients with stable vns therapy (age: 45 ± 10 yrs; body mass index; 25.2 ± 3.5 kg/m(2)) were included between January 2011 and June 2012. Ten subjects were measured twice, once with active and once with inactivated VNS. Five other subjects were measured twice, once with active VNS at room temperature and once with active VNS under cold exposure in order to determine maximal cold-induced BAT activity. BAT activity was assessed by 18-Fluoro-Deoxy-Glucose-Positron-Emission-Tomography-and-Computed-Tomography. Basal metabolic rate (BMR) was significantly higher when VNS was turned on (mean change; $+2.2\%$). Mean BAT activity was not significantly different between active VNS and inactive VNS (BAT SUV(Mean); 0.55 ± 0.25 versus 0.67 ± 0.46, $P = 0.619$). However, the change in energy expenditure upon VNS intervention (On-Off) was significantly correlated to the change in BAT activity ($r = 0.935$, $P<0.001$). **CONCLUSIONS:** VNS significantly increases energy expenditure. The observed change in energy expenditure was significantly related to the change in BAT activity. This suggests a role for BAT in the VNS increase in energy expenditure. Chronic VNS may have a beneficial effect on the human energy balance that has potential application for weight management therapy.

Reducing White Fat with Arginine

FREE FULLTEXT
Source: Front Biosci (Landmark Ed). 2012 Jun
1;17:2237-46.
Title: Regulatory roles for L-arginine in reducing
white adipose tissue.

Authors:Tan B, Li X, Yin Y, Wu Z, Liu C, Tekwe
CD, Wu G.

Abstract: As the nitrogenous precursor of nitric
oxide, L-arginine regulates multiple metabolic pathways involved in the metabolism of fatty acids, glucose, amino acids, and proteins through cell signaling
and gene expression. Specifically, arginine stimulates
lipolysis and the expression of key genes responsible
for activation of fatty acid oxidation to CO_2 and
water. The underlying mechanisms involve increases
in the expression of peroxisome proliferator-activated
receptor-gamma coactivator-1 alpha (PGC-1 alpha),
mitochondrial biogenesis, and the growth of brown
adipose tissue growth. Furthermore, arginine regulates adipocyte-muscle crosstalk and energy partitioning via the secretion of cytokines and hormones.
In addition, arginine enhances AMP-activated protein kinase (AMPK) expression and activity, thereby
modulating lipid metabolism and energy balance
toward the loss of triacylglycerols. **Growing evidence
shows that dietary supplementation with arginine
effectively reduces white adipose tissue in Zucker
diabetic fatty rats, diet-induced obese rats, grow-
ing-finishing pigs, and obese patients with type
II diabetes. Thus, arginine can be used to prevent
and treat adiposity and the associated metabolic
syndrome.**

Walking and Bicycling

FREE FULLTEXT
Source: Acta Médica Portuguesa. Nov-Dec 2011.
Title: [Physical activity and public health: recommendations for exercise prescription].
[Article in Portuguese]

Authors: Mendes R, Sousa N, Barata JL.

Abstract: During the last half century scientific data have been accumulated, through epidemiological and clinical studies that clearly document the significant health benefits associated with regular physical activity. This paper will analyse the latest recommendations for prescribing exercise in all age groups in healthy subjects and to individuals with chronic non-communicable diseases such as overweight, obesity, diabetes, hypertension, atherosclerotic cardiovascular disease and cancer, that contribute to the leading causes of global mortality. A search in the Pubmed database was performed and were also searched the recommendations of the World Health Organization and scientific organizations in Portugal. **Most health benefits occur with at least 150 minutes of aerobic exercise of moderate intensity, accumulated over the week, which can be split into periods of at least 10 minutes.** *Brisk walking seems to be the preferred aerobic exercise. Vigorous intensity aerobic exercise and resistance exercises for muscle strengthening, at least two days a week are also recommended. Children, youth, older adults and people with overweight have particular needs for physical activity.* Additional benefits occur with increasing quantity and quality of physical activity through the proper manipulation of the exercise density (intensity, frequency and duration). However, some physical activity is better than none. The role of health professionals in prescribing appropriate exercise to their patients is fundamental to their involvement in increasing their physical activity levels and thus contributing to their health promotion and prevention and treatment of major noncommunicable chronic diseases.

Is Sitting at Your Computer Killing You?

FREE FULLTEXT
Source: Prev Med. 2015 Jul;76:92-102. doi: 10.1016/j.ypmed.2015.04.013. Epub 2015 Apr 23.
Title: Accelerometer-measured sedentary time and cardiometabolic biomarkers: A systematic review.
Authors: Brocklebank LA, Falconer CL, Page AS, Perry R, Cooper AR.

Abstract: OBJECTIVE: We conducted a systematic review to investigate the cross-sectional and prospective associations of accelerometer-measured total sedentary time and breaks in sedentary time with individual cardiometabolic biomarkers in adults ≥18 years of age.
METHODS: Ovid Medline, Embase, Web of Science and the Cochrane Library were searched for studies meeting the inclusion criteria. Due to inconsistencies in the measurement and analysis of sedentary time, data was synthesised and presented narratively rather than as a meta-analysis.
RESULTS: Twenty-nine studies were included in the review; twenty-eight reported on total sedentary time and six on breaks in sedentary time. There was consistent evidence from cross-sectional data of an unfavourable association between total sedentary

118

time and insulin sensitivity. There was also some evidence that total sedentary time was unfavourably associated with fasting insulin, insulin resistance and triglycerides. Furthermore, there was some evidence from cross-sectional data of a favourable association between breaks in sedentary time and triglycerides. CONCLUSION: **Total sedentary time was consistently shown to be associated with poorer insulin sensitivity, even after adjusting for time spent in physical activity. This finding supports the proposed association between sedentary time and the development of Type 2 diabetes and reinforces the need to identify interventions to reduce time spent sedentary.**

The Possible Benefits of Standing Desks

FREE FULLTEXT
Source: Int J Environ Res Public Health. 2014 Sep 10;11(9):9361-75. doi: 10.3390/ijerph110909361.
Title: The evaluation of the impact of a stand-biased desk on energy expenditure and physical activity for elementary school students.
Authors: Benden ME, Zhao H, Jeffrey CE, Wendel ML, Blake JJ.
Abstract: Due to the increasing prevalence of childhood obesity, the association between classroom furniture and energy expenditure as well as physical activity was examined using a standing-desk intervention in three central-Texas elementary schools. Of the 480 students in the 24 classrooms randomly assigned to either a seated or stand-biased desk

equipped classroom, 374 agreed to participate in a week-long data collection during the fall and spring semesters. Each participant's data was collected using Sensewear® armbands and was comprised of measures of energy expenditure (EE) and step count. A hierarchical linear mixed effects model showed that children in seated desk classrooms had significantly lower (EE) and fewer steps during the standardized lecture time than children in stand-biased classrooms after adjusting for grade, race, and gender. **The use of a standing desk showed a significant higher mean energy expenditure by 0.16 kcal/min (p < 0.0001) in the fall semester, and a higher EE by 0.08 kcal/min (p = 0.0092) in the spring semester.**

Yoga and Weight Loss

FREE FULLTEXT
Source: BMC Complement Altern Med. 2014 Jul 1;14:212. doi: 10.1186/1472-6882-14-212.
Title: A yoga intervention for type 2 diabetes risk reduction: a pilot randomized controlled trial.
Authors: McDermott KA1, Rao MR, Nagarathna R, Murphy EJ, Burke A, Nagendra RH, Hecht FM.

Abstract : BACKGROUND: Type 2 diabetes is a major health problem in many countries including India. Yoga may be an effective type 2 diabetes prevention strategy in India, particularly given its cultural familiarity.
METHODS: This was a parallel, randomized controlled pilot study to collect feasibility and pre-

liminary efficacy data on yoga for diabetes risk factors among people at high risk of diabetes. Primary outcomes included: changes in BMI, waist circumference, fasting blood glucose, postprandial blood glucose, insulin, insulin resistance, blood pressure, and cholesterol. We also looked at measures of psychological well-being including changes in depression, anxiety, positive and negative affect and perceived stress. Forty-one participants with elevated fasting blood glucose in Bangalore, India were randomized to either yoga (n = 21) or a walking control (n = 20). Participants were asked to either attend yoga classes or complete monitored walking 3-6 days per week for eight weeks. Randomization and allocation was performed using computer-generated random numbers and group assignments delivered in sealed, opaque envelopes generated by off-site study staff. Data were analyzed based on intention to treat.

RESULTS: This study was feasible in terms of recruitment, retention and adherence. In addition, yoga participants had significantly greater reductions in weight, waist circumference and BMI versus control (weight -0.8 ± 2.1 vs. 1.4 ± 3.6, p = 0.02; waist circumference -4.2 ± 4.8 vs. 0.7 ± 4.2, p < 0.01; BMI -0.2 ± 0.8 vs. 0.6 ± 1.6, p = 0.05). There were no between group differences in fasting blood glucose, postprandial blood glucose, insulin resistance or any other factors related to diabetes risk or psychological well-being. There were significant reductions in systolic and diastolic blood pressure, total cholesterol, anxiety, depression, negative affect and perceived stress in both the yoga intervention and walking control over the course of the study.

CONCLUSION: Among Indians with elevated fasting blood glucose, we found that participation in an 8-week yoga intervention was feasible and

resulted in greater weight loss and reduction in waist circumference when compared to a walking control. Yoga offers a promising lifestyle intervention for decreasing weight-related type 2 diabetes risk factors and potentially increasing psychological well-being.

Mindful Eating and Weight Loss

Source: Health Educ Behav. 2014 Apr;41(2):145-54. doi: 10.1177/1090198113493092. Epub 2013 Jul 12.
Title: Comparison of a mindful eating intervention to a diabetes self-management intervention among adults with type 2 diabetes: a randomized controlled trial.
Authors: Miller CK, Kristeller JL, Headings A, Nagaraja H.
Abstract Mindful eating may be an effective intervention for increasing awareness of hunger and satiety cues, improving eating regulation and dietary patterns, reducing symptoms of depression and anxiety, and promoting weight loss. Diabetes self-management education (DSME), which addresses knowledge, self-efficacy, and outcome expectations for improving food choices, also may be an effective intervention for diabetes self-care. Yet few studies have compared the impact of mindful eating to a DSME-based treatment approach on patient outcomes. Adults 35 to 65 years old with type 2 diabetes for ≥1 year not requiring insulin therapy were re-

cruited from the community and randomly assigned to treatment group. The impact of a group-based 3-month mindful eating intervention (MB-EAT-D; n = 27) to a group-based 3-month DSME "Smart Choices" (SC) intervention (n = 25) post-intervention and at 3-month follow-up was evaluated. Repeated-measures ANOVA with contrast analysis compared change in outcomes across time. There was no significant difference between groups in weight change. Significant improvement in depressive symptoms, outcome expectations, nutrition and eating-related self-efficacy, and cognitive control and disinhibition of control regarding eating behaviors occurred for both groups (all $p < .0125$) at 3-month follow-up. The SC group had greater increase in nutrition knowledge and self-efficacy than the MB-EAT-D group (all $p < .05$) at 3-month follow-up. **MB-EAT-D had significant increase in mindfulness, whereas the SC group had significant increase in fruit and vegetable consumption at study end (all $p < .0125$). Both SC and MB-EAT-D were effective treatments for diabetes self-management.** The availability of mindful eating and DSME-based approaches offers patients greater choices in meeting their self-care needs.

Long Term Meditation and Yoga and Basal Metabolic Rate

There seems to be a point of diminishing returns when it comes to yoga and meditation weight-wise, at least.

FREE FULLTEXT

Source: BMC Complement Altern Med. 2006 Aug 31;6:28.
Title: The effect of long term combined yoga practice on the basal metabolic rate of healthy adults.
Authors: Chaya MS, Kurpad AV, Nagendra HR, Nagarathna R.

Abstract BACKGROUND: Different procedures practiced in yoga have stimulatory or inhibitory effects on the basal metabolic rate when studied acutely. In daily life however, these procedures are usually practiced in combination. The purpose of the present study was to investigate the net change in the basal metabolic rate (BMR) of individuals actively engaging in a combination of yoga practices (asana or yogic postures, meditation and pranayama or breathing exercises) for a minimum period of six months, at a residential yoga education and research center at Bangalore. **METHODS:** The measured BMR of individuals practicing yoga through a combination of practices was compared with that of control subjects who did not practice yoga but led similar lifestyles. **RESULTS:** The BMR of the yoga practitioners was significantly lower than that of the non-yoga group, and was lower by about 13 % when adjusted for body weight (P < 0.001). This difference persisted when the groups were stratified by gender; however, the difference in BMR adjusted for body weight was greater in women than men (about 8 and 18% respectively). In addition, the mean BMR of the yoga group was significantly lower than their predicted values, while the mean BMR of non-yoga group was comparable with their predicted values derived from 1985 WHO/FAO/UNU predictive equations. **CONCLUSION: This study shows that there is a significantly reduced BMR, probably linked to reduced arousal, with the long term practice of yoga**

using a combination of stimulatory and inhibitory yogic practices.

Thirty Minutes of Exercise Enough to Strengthen The Body on a Cellular Level

<u>FREE FULLTEXT</u>
Source: PLoS One. 2014 Apr 21;9(4):e92088. doi: 10.1371/journal.pone.0092088. eCollection 2014.
Title: Acute exercise leads to regulation of telomere-associated genes and microRNA expression in immune cells.
Authors: Chilton WL, Marques FZ, West J, Kannourakis G, Berzins SP, O'Brien BJ, Charchar FJ.
Abstract: Telomeres are specialized nucleoprotein structures that protect chromosomal ends from degradation. These structures progressively shorten during cellular division and can signal replicative senescence below a critical length. Telomere length is predominantly maintained by the enzyme telomerase. **Significant decreases in telomere length and telomerase activity are associated with a host of chronic diseases; conversely their maintenance underpins the optimal function of the adaptive immune system. Habitual physical activity is associated with longer leukocyte telomere length; however, the precise mechanisms are unclear.** Potential hypotheses include regulation of telomeric gene transcription and/or microRNAs (miRNAs). We investigated the acute exercise-induced response of telomeric genes and miRNAs in twenty-two healthy males (mean age=24.1±1.55 years). Partici-

pants undertook 30 minutes of treadmill running at 80% of peak oxygen uptake. Blood samples were taken before exercise, immediately post-exercise and 60 minutes post-exercise. Total RNA from white blood cells was submitted to miRNA arrays and telomere extension mRNA array. Results were individually validated in white blood cells and sorted T cell lymphocyte subsets using quantitative real-time PCR (qPCR). Telomerase reverse transcriptase (TERT) mRNA (P=0.001) and sirtuin-6 (SIRT6) (P<0.05) mRNA expression were upregulated in white blood cells after exercise. Fifty-six miRNAs were also differentially regulated post-exercise (FDR <0.05). In silico analysis identified four miRNAs (miR-186, miR-181, miR-15a and miR-96) that potentially targeted telomeric gene mRNA. The four miRNAs exhibited significant upregulation 60 minutes post-exercise (P<0.001). Telomeric repeat binding factor 2, interacting protein (TERF2IP) was identified as a potential binding target for miR-186 and miR-96 and demonstrated concomitant downregulation (P<0.01) at the corresponding time point. Intense cardiorespiratory exercise was sufficient to differentially regulate key telomeric genes and miRNAs in white blood cells. These results may provide a mechanistic insight into telomere homeostasis and improved immune function and physical health.

Other Aspects of Weight Management that are Important but Often Overlooked
Complementary and Alternative Traditional Treatments (CAM) of High Blood Sugar

FREE FULLTEXT
Source: Nutr J. 2014; 13: 102. Published online
2014 Oct 21. doi: 10.1186/1475-2891-13-102
PMCID: PMC4210501
Title: The use of Complementary and Alternative
Medicines (CAMs) in the treatment of diabetes mellitus: is continued use safe and effective?
Authors: Medagama AB, Bandara R.
Abstract: Diabetes mellitus is a major cause of morbidity and mortality worldwide, with a prevalence of
347 million in 2013. Complementary and Alternative Medicines (CAM) are a group of remedies that
is fast gaining acceptance among individuals. Cinnamon, Bitter gourd (Momordica charantia) and Fenugreek (Trigonella foenum-graecum) are 3 widely used
CAMs used worldwide for the treatment of diabetes.
Data on safety and efficacy is limited, but the consumption is wide. Crepe ginger (Costus speciosus)
and Ivy gourd (Coccinia grandis) are 2 plants used
widely in the Asian region for their presumed hypo-
glycaemic properties.

Apps and Weight Loss

FREE FULLTEXT
Source: Int J Behav Nutr Phys Act. 2016 Mar
10;13(1):35. doi: 10.1186/s12966-016-0359-9.
Title: A review and content analysis of engagement,
functionality, aesthetics, information quality, and
change techniques in the most popular commercial
apps for weight management.
Authors: Bardus M, van Beurden SB, Smith JR,

Abraham C.

Abstract: BACKGROUND: There are thousands
of apps promoting dietary improvement, increased
physical activity (PA) and weight management. Despite a growing number of reviews in this area, popular apps have not been comprehensively analysed in
terms of features related to engagement, functionality, aesthetics, information quality, and content,
including the types of change techniques employed.
METHODS: The databases containing information
about all Health and Fitness apps on GP and iTunes
(7,954 and 25,491 apps) were downloaded in April
2015. Database filters were applied to select the most
popular apps available in both stores. Two researchers screened the descriptions selecting only weight
management apps. Features, app quality and content
were independently assessed using the Mobile App
Rating Scale (MARS) and previously-defined categories of techniques relevant to behaviour change.
Inter-coder reliabilities were calculated, and correlations between features explored.
RESULTS: Of the 23 popular apps included in the
review 16 were free (70 %), 15 (65 %) addressed
weight control, diet and PA combined; 19 (83 %)
allowed behavioural tracking. On 5-point MARS
scales, apps were of average quality (Md = 3.2,
IQR = 1.4); "functionality" (Md = 4.0, IQR = 1.1)
was the highest and "information quality" (Md = 2.0,
IQR = 1.1) was the lowest domain. On average, 10
techniques were identified per app (range: 1-17)
and of the 34 categories applied, goal setting and
self-monitoring techniques were most frequently
identified. App quality was positively correlated with
number of techniques included (rho = .58, p < .01)
and number of "technical" features (rho = .48,
p < .05), which was also associated with the number
128

of techniques included (rho = .61, p < .01). Apps that provided tracking used significantly more techniques than those that did not. Apps with automated tracking scored significantly higher in engagement, aesthetics, and overall MARS scores. Those that used change techniques previously associated with effectiveness (i.e., goal setting, self-monitoring and feedback) also had better "information quality".

CONCLUSIONS: **Popular apps assessed have overall moderate quality and include behavioural tracking features and a range of change techniques associated with behaviour change. These apps may influence behaviour, although more attention to information quality and evidence-based content are warranted to improve their quality.**

Belief in God Protects the Faithful

A little faith never hurt anyone.

Source: J Relig Health. 2013 Mar;52(1):91-106.
Title: Review of clinical medicine and religious practice.
Authors: Stewart WC, Adams MP, Stewart JA, Nelson LA.
Abstract: The purpose was to evaluate faith-based studies within the medical literature to determine whether there are ways to help physicians understand how religion affects patients' lives and diseases. We reviewed articles that assessed the influence of religious practices on medicine as a primary or secondary variable in clinical practice. This review evaluated 49 articles and found that religious faith is important to many patients, particularly those with serious dis-

ease, and patients depend on it as a positive coping mechanism. The findings of this review can suggest that patients frequently practice religion and interact with God about their disease state. This spiritual interaction may benefit the patient by providing comfort, increasing knowledge about their disease, greater treatment adherence, and quality of life. **The results of prayer on specific disease states appear inconsistent with cardiovascular disease but stronger in other disease states.**

A Glass of Alcohol Daily will give you a longer, healthier life

If you are a compulsive, addictive type, I would steer clear of drinking because it could easily get out of hand; however, if you can limit yourself to a glass of red wine daily, you'll probably add healthy years to your life.

FREE FULLTEXT
Source:Nutrients. 2012 Jul;4(7):759-81. doi: 10.3390/nu4070759. Epub 2012 Jul 10.
Title: Wine, beer, alcohol and polyphenols on cardiovascular disease and cancer.
Authors: Arranz S, Chiva-Blanch G, Valderas-Martínez P, Medina-Remón A, Lamuela-Raventós RM, Estruch R.

Abstract: Since ancient times, people have attributed a variety of health benefits to moderate consumption of fermented beverages such as wine and beer, often without any scientific basis. There is evidence that excessive or binge alcohol consumption is associated with increased morbidity and mortality, as well as with work related and traffic accidents. On the contrary, at the moment, several epidemiological studies have suggested that moderate consumption of alcohol reduces overall mortality, mainly from coronary diseases. However, there are discrepancies regarding the specific effects of different types of beverages (wine, beer and spirits) on the cardiovascular system and cancer, and also whether the possible protective effects of alcoholic beverages are due to their alcoholic content (ethanol) or to their non-alcoholic components (mainly polyphenols). Epidemiological and clinical studies have pointed out that regular and moderate wine consumption (one to two glasses a day) is associated with decreased incidence of cardiovascular disease (CVD), hypertension, diabetes, and certain types of cancer, including colon, basal cell, ovarian, and prostate carcinoma. Moderate beer consumption has also been associated with these effects, but to a lesser degree, probably because of beer's lower phenolic content. These health benefits have mainly been attributed to an increase in antioxidant capacity, changes in lipid profiles, and the anti-inflammatory effects produced by these alcoholic beverages. **This review summarizes the main protective effects on the cardiovascular system and cancer resulting from moderate wine and beer intake due mainly to their common components, alcohol and polyphenols.**

Living in Polluted Cities can Cause Asthma, Liver and Heart Damage

Why not live in the countryside if you have a chance, or at least get away to the countryside when you get a chance?

FREE FULLTEXT
Source: Toxicol Res. 2014 Jun;30(2):65-70. doi: 10.5487/TR.2014.30.2.065.
Title: The role of air pollutants in initiating liver disease.

Authors: Kim JW, Park S, Lim CW, Lee K, Kim B.

Abstract: Recent episodes of severe air pollution in eastern Asia have been reported in the scientific literature and news media. Therefore, there is growing concern about the systemic effects of air pollution on human health. **Along with the other well-known harmful effects of air pollution, recently, several animal models have provided strong evidence that air pollutants can induce liver toxicity and act to accelerate liver inflammation and steatosis.** This review briefly describes examples where exposure to air pollutants was involved in liver toxicity, focusing on how particulate matter (PM) or carbon black (CB) may be translocated from lung to liver and what liver diseases are closely associated with these air pollutants.

Neighborhood Planning, Walking, and Better Health

FREE FULLTEXT

Source: BMC Public Health. 2015 Aug 11;15:768.
doi: 10.1186/s12889-015-2082-x.
Title: Associations between neighbourhood walkability and daily steps in adults: a systematic review and meta-analysis.
Authors: Hajna S, Ross NA, Brazeau AS, Bélisle P, Joseph L, Dasgupta K.
Abstract: **BACKGROUND:** Higher street connectivity, land use mix and residential density (collectively referred to as neighbourhood walkability) have been linked to higher levels of walking. The objective of our study was to summarize the current body of knowledge on the association between neighbourhood walkability and biosensor-assessed daily steps in adults.

METHODS: We conducted a systematic search of PubMed, SCOPUS, and Embase (Ovid) for articles published prior to May 2014 on the association between walkability (based on Geographic Information Systems-derived street connectivity, land use mix, and/or residential density) and daily steps (pedometer or accelerometer-assessed) in adults. The mean differences in daily steps between adults living in high versus low walkable neighbourhoods were pooled across studies using a Bayesian hierarchical model. **RESULTS:** The search strategy yielded 8,744 unique abstracts. Thirty of these underwent full article review of which six met the inclusion criteria. Four of these studies were conducted in Europe and two were conducted in Asia. A meta-analysis of four of these six studies indicates that participants living in high compared to low walkable neighbourhoods accumulate 766 more steps per day (95 % credible interval 250, 1271). This accounts for approximately 8 % of recommended daily steps. **CONCLUSIONS: The results of European and**

Asian studies support the hypothesis that higher neighbourhood walkability is associated with higher levels of biosensor-assessed walking in adults. More studies on this association are needed in North America.

Working at Night and Weight Loss Difficulty

It turns out that people who stay up late for work or study for even one day are dysregulating their metabolism to make it harder to maintain a healthy weight, mostly due to an increase of the hunger hormone ghrelin in the brain and body.

Source: Proc Natl Acad Sci U S A. 2014 Dec 2;111(48):17302-7. doi: 10.1073/pnas.1412021111. Epub 2014 Nov 17.
Title: Impact of circadian misalignment on energy metabolism during simulated nightshift work.
Authors: McHill AW, Melanson E, Higgins J, Connick E, Moehlman TM, Stothard ER, Wright KP Jr.
Abstract **Eating at a time when the internal circadian clock promotes sleep is a novel risk factor for weight gain and obesity, yet little is known about mechanisms by which circadian misalignment leads to metabolic dysregulation in humans.** We studied 14 adults in a 6-d inpatient simulated shiftwork protocol and quantified changes in energy expenditure, macronutrient utilization, appetitive hormones, sleep, and circadian phase during day versus nightshift work. We found that total daily energy expenditure increased by 4% on the transition day to
134

the first nightshift, which consisted of an afternoon nap and extended wakefulness, whereas total daily energy expenditure decreased by 3% on each of the second and third nightshift days, which consisted of daytime sleep followed by afternoon and nighttime wakefulness. Contrary to expectations, energy expenditure decreased by 12-16% during scheduled daytime sleep opportunities despite disturbed sleep. The thermic effect of feeding also decreased in response to a late dinner on the first nightshift. Total daily fat utilization increased on the first and second nightshift days, contrary to expectations, and carbohydrate and protein utilization were reduced on the second nightshift day. Ratings of hunger were decreased during nightshift days despite decreases in 24-h levels of the satiety hormones leptin and peptide-YY. Findings suggest that reduced total daily energy expenditure during nightshift schedules and reduced energy expenditure in response to dinner represent contributing mechanisms by which humans working and eating during the biological night, when the circadian clock is promoting sleep, may increase the risk of weight gain and obesity.

Neurobiol Dis. 2013 Oct;58:169-78. doi: 10.1016/j.nbd.2013.05.003. Epub 2013 May 16.

Sunlight AND Weight

FREE FULLTEXT
Source: Indian J Endocrinol Metab. 2014 Nov;18(Suppl 1):S9-S16. doi: 10.4103/2230-8210.145043.
Title: Vitamin D deficiency in adolescents.

Authors: Soliman AT, De Sanctis V, Elalaily R, Bedair S, Kassem I.

Abstract: The prevalence of severe vitamin D deficiency (VDD) in adolescents is variable but considerably high in many countries, especially in Middle-east and Southeast Asia. Different factors attribute to this deficiency including lack of sunlight exposure due to cultural dress codes and veiling or due to pigmented skin, and less time spent outdoors, because of hot weather, and lower vitamin D intake. A potent adaptation process significantly modifies the clinical presentation and therefore clinical presentations may be subtle and go unnoticed, thus making true prevalence studies difficult. Adolescents with severe VDD may present with vague manifestations including pain in weight-bearing joints, back, thighs and/or calves, difficulty in walking and/or climbing stairs, or running and muscle cramps. Adaptation includes increased parathormone (PTH) and decreased insulin-like growth factor-I (IGF-I) secretion. PTH enhances the tubular reabsorption of Ca and stimulates the kidneys to produce 1, 25-(OH) 2D3 that increases intestinal calcium absorption and dissolves the mineralized collagen matrix in bone, causing osteopenia and osteoporosis to provide enough Ca to prevent hypocalcaemia. Decreased insulin like growth factor-I (IGF-I) delays bone growth to economize calcium consumption. Radiological changes are not uncommon and include osteoporosis/osteopenia affecting long bones as well as vertebrae and ribs, bone cysts, decalcification of the metaphysis of the long bones and pseudo fractures. In severe cases pathological fractures and deformities may occur. Vitamin D treatment of adolescents with VDD differs considerably in different studies and proved to be effective in treating all clinical, biochemical, and radiological manifestations. Different treatment regimens for VDD have been discussed and presented in this mini-review for practical use. Adequate vitamin D replacement after treating VDD, improving calcium intake (milk and dairy products), encouraging adequate exposure to the sun and possible enrichment of the stable food with vitamin D in areas with high prevalence of VDD are important measures to prevent the harmful consequences of VDD.

Neurobiology of Sweet Food

It seems that the craving for sweet foods and drinks is a vicious cycle. The more sweet foodstuffs we have, the more we crave them.

FREE FULLTEXT
Source: Yale J Biol Med. 2010 Jun;83(2):101-8.
Title: Gain weight by "going diet?" Artificial sweeteners and the neurobiology of sugar cravings: Neuroscience 2010.
Author: Yang Q

Abstract: America's obesity epidemic has gathered much media attention recently. A rise in the percent of the population who are obese coincides with an increase in the widespread use of non-caloric artificial sweeteners, such as aspartame (e.g., Diet Coke) and sucralose (e.g., Pepsi One), in food products (Figure 1). Both forward and reverse causalities have been proposed. While people often choose "diet" or "light" products to lose weight, research studies suggest that artificial sweeteners may contribute to weight gain. In this mini-review, inspired by a discussion with Dr. Dana Small at Yale's Neuroscience 2010 conference in April, I first examine the development of artificial sweeteners in a historic context. I then summarize the epidemiological and experimental evidence concerning their effects on weight. Finally, I attempt to explain those effects in light of the neurobiology of food reward.

Acupuncture for Weight Management

FREE FULLTEXT
Source: J Tradit Chin Med. 2008 Jun;28(2):139-47.
Title: A clinical survey of acupuncture slimming.
Author: Zhang X
Abstract: Acupuncture is affirmatively effective in treating obesity with its flexible point selection and various methods without toxic and side effects. This review will focus on different therapeutic methods and academic thoughts in acupuncture slimming and evaluate its current state and prospect.

Stevia: Actually, A Good Sweetener?

FREE FULLTEXT
Source: Molecules. 2015 Dec 26;21(1). pii: E38. doi: 10.3390/molecules21010038.
Title: Is Stevia rebaudiana Bertoni a Non Cariogenic Sweetener? A Review\

Authors: Ferrazzano GF, Cantile T, Alcidi B, Coda M, Ingenito A, Zarrelli A,, Di Fabio G, Pollio A.

Abstract: Stevia rebaudiana Bertoni is a small perennial shrub of the Asteraceae (Compositae) family that is native to South America, particularly Brazil and Paraguay, where it is known as "stevia" or "honey leaf" for its powerful sweetness. **Several studies have suggested that in addition to their sweetness, steviosides and their related compounds, including rebaudioside A and isosteviol, may offer additional therapeutic benefits. These benefits include anti-hyperglycaemic, anti-hypertensive, anti-inflammatory, anti-tumor, anti-diarrheal, diuretic, and immunomodulatory actions. Additionally, critical analysis of the literature supports the anti-bacterial role of steviosides on oral bacteria flora.** The aim of this review is to show the emerging results regarding the anti-cariogenic properties of S. rebaudiana Bertoni. Data shown in the present paper provide evidence that stevioside extracts from S. rebaudiana are not cariogenic. Future research should be focused on in vivo studies to evaluate the effects on dental caries of regular consumption of S. rebaudiana extract-based products.

Breakfast: Skip it and Gain Weight

Source: Obes Res Clin Pract. 2014 May-Jun;8(3):e201-98. doi: 10.1016/j.orcp.2013.01.001.
Title: Effect of breakfast skipping on diurnal variation of energy metabolism and blood glucose.

Authors: Kobayashi F, Ogata H, Omi N, Nagasaka S, Yamaguchi S, Hibi M, Tokuyama K.

Abstract: Epidemiological studies suggest an association between breakfast skipping and body weight gain, insulin resistance or type 2 diabetes. Time when meal is consumed affects postprandial increase in energy expenditure and blood glucose, and breakfast skipping may reduce 24 h energy expenditure and elevate blood glucose level. The present study evaluated the effect of breakfast skipping on diurnal variation of energy metabolism and blood glucose. **The skipped breakfast was compensated by following big meals at lunch and supper.** In a randomized repeated-measure design with or without breakfast, eight males stayed twice in a room-size respiratory chamber. Blood glucose was recorded with a continuous glucose monitoring system. Breakfast skipping did not affect 24 h energy expenditure, fat oxidation and thermic effect of food, but increased overall 24 h average of blood glucose (83 ± 3 vs 89 ± 2 mg/dl, $P < 0.05$). Unlike 24 h glucose level, 24 h energy expenditure was robust when challenged by breakfast skipping. These observations suggest that changes in glucose homeostasis precede that of energy balance, in the potential sequence caused by breakfast skipping, if this dietary habit has any effect on energy balance.

Portion Control and Weight Loss

FULL FULLTEXT
Source: Int J Obes (Lond). 2014 Jul;38 Suppl 1:S1-8. doi: 10.1038/ijo.2014.82.

140

Title: What is the role of portion control in weight management?

Author: Rolls BJ.

Abstract: Systematic studies have shown that providing individuals with larger portions of foods and beverages leads to substantial increases in energy intake. The effect is sustained over weeks, supporting the possibility that large portions have a role in the development of obesity. The challenge is to find strategies to effectively manage the effects of portion size. One approach involves teaching people to select appropriate portions and to use tools that facilitate portion control. Although tools such as portion-control plates have been shown in several randomized trials to improve weight loss, limited data are available on whether education and tools lead to long-term changes in eating behavior and body weight. Another approach is to use pre-portioned foods (PPFs) to add structure to meals and minimize decisions about the amount of food to eat. A number of randomized controlled trials have demonstrated the efficacy of both liquid meal replacements and solid PPFs for weight loss and weight loss maintenance, but it is not known if they lead to better understanding of appropriate portions. **Although portion control is important for weight management, urging people simply to 'eat less' of all foods may not be the best approach as high-energy-dense foods disproportionately increase energy intake compared with those lower in energy density. A more effective strategy may be to encourage people to increase the proportion of foods low in energy density in their diets while limiting portions of high-energy-dense foods. If people lower the energy density of their diet, they can eat satisfying portions while managing their body weight.**

Mind over Belly

FREE FULLTEXT
Source: Int J Obes (Lond). 2014 Jul;38 Suppl 1:S9-12. doi: 10.1038/ijo.2014.83.
Title: Mind over platter: pre-meal planning and the control of meal size in humans.
Author: Brunstrom JM.
Abstract: It is widely accepted that meal size is governed by psychological and physiological processes that generate fullness towards the end of a meal. However, observations of natural eating behaviour suggest that this preoccupation with within-meal events may be misplaced and that the role of immediate post-ingestive feedback (for example, gastric stretch) has been overstated. This review considers the proposition that the locus of control is more likely to be expressed in decisions about portion size, before a meal begins. Consistent with this idea, we have discovered that people are extremely adept at estimating the 'expected satiety' and 'expected satiation' of different foods. These expectations are learned over time and they are highly correlated with the number of calories that end up on our plate. Indeed, across a range of foods, the large variation in expected satiety/satiation may be a more important determinant of meal size than relatively subtle differences in palatability. Building on related advances, it would also appear that memory for portion size has an important role in generating satiety after a meal has been consumed. Together, these findings expose the importance of planning and episodic memory in the control of appetite and food intake in humans.

The Autonomic Nervous System and Weight

FREE FULLTEXT
Front Physiol. 2015 Aug 25;6:234. doi: 10.3389/fphys.2015.00234. eCollection 2015.

Title: Does the sympathetic nervous system contribute to the pathophysiology of metabolic syndrome?

Authors: Moreira MC, Pinto IS, Mourão AA, Fajemiroye JO, Colombari E, Reis ÂA, Freiria-Oliveira AH, Ferreira-Neto ML, Pedrino GR.

Abstract: The metabolic syndrome (MS), formally known as syndrome X, is a clustering of several risk factors such as obesity, hypertension, insulin resistance, and dyslipidemia which could lead to the development of diabetes and cardiovascular diseases (CVD). The frequent changes in the definition and diagnostic criteria of MS are indications of the controversy and the challenges surrounding the understanding of this syndrome among researchers. Obesity and insulin resistance are leading risk factors of MS. Moreover, obesity and hypertension are closely associated to the increase and aggravation of oxidative stress. The recommended treatment of MS frequently involves change of lifestyles to prevent weight gain. **MS is not only an important screening tool for the identification of individuals at high risk of CVD and diabetes but also an indicator of suitable treatment. As sympathetic disturbances and oxidative stress are often associated with obesity and hypertension, the present review summarizes the role of sympathetic nervous system and oxidative stress in the Metabolic Syndrome.**

Protein and Weight Control in Diabetes

FREE FULLTEXT
Source: J Nutr. 2015 Jan;145(1):164S-169S. doi:
10.3945/jn.114.194878. Epub 2014 Dec 3.
Title: Dietary protein is important in the practical
management of prediabetes and type 2 diabetes.
Authors: Campbell AP, Rains TM.
Abstract: Many misconceptions surround the role
of dietary protein in the management of diabetes.
Although dietary recommendations for managing
diabetes have changed greatly over the centuries,
recommended protein intake has remained relatively
constant. Currently, recommendations for protein
intake are based on individual assessment and the
consideration of other health issues and implications, such as the extent of glycemic control, the
presence of kidney disease, overweight and obesity,
and the age of the patient. Two common misconceptions about dietary protein in diabetes management
are that a certain amount of the protein consumed
is converted into blood glucose and that consuming too much protein can lead to diabetic kidney
disease. These misconceptions have been disproven.
**For many people with type 2 diabetes, aiming
for 20-30% of total energy intake as protein is
the goal. Exceptions may be for those individuals with impaired renal function. A protein intake
of this amount can be beneficial by improving
glycemic control, aiding in satiety and preserva-
tion of lean body mass during weight loss in those
with both diabetes and prediabetes, and providing for the increased protein requirements of the
older adult.** Health care providers should discuss the
role of dietary protein with their patients, reinforce
sources of protein in the diet, and use simple but

effective teaching tools, such as the plate method, to convey important nutrition messages. In addition, health care providers should recognize that persons with diabetes are attempting to manage many other aspects of their diabetes, including blood glucose monitoring, physical activity, taking of medication, risk reduction, and problem solving.

Fat and Obesity

FREE FULLTEXT
Title: Food Intake and Obesity: The Case of Fat.
Source: Fat Detection: Taste, Texture, and Post Ingestive Effects. Boca Raton (FL): CRC Press/Taylor & Francis; 2010. Chapter 22. Frontiers in Neuroscience.
Authors: Smilowitz JT, German JB, Zivkovic AM.
Excerpt: Studies that simultaneously quantify the lipid metabolites—substrates and products of biochemical pathways—in tissues and biofluids have proven to be extremely valuable in revealing dysregulation in biochemical pathways associated with other metabolic diseases such as atherosclerosis. This chapter describes the use of comprehensive analysis of lipids associated with various biochemical pathways combined with specific dietary challenges to reveal the dynamic nature of an individual's metabolic phenotype (German et al., 2007). Circulating lipids are derived from both diet and endogenous metabolism. These lipids are highly dynamic, interactive biological molecules that make up most cellular components and signaling molecules, and they dic-

tate energy partitioning and control of food intake. Remarkably, although food intake is central to the problem of obesity, the vast majority of studies attempting to explain the variations in metabolism that could account for excess intake and for its metabolic consequences have examined individuals and their various physiological, metabolic, and endocrine characteristics in the fasted condition. Furthermore, studies to date have examined only a subset of the metabolites representing the various biochemical pathways that are both responsive to dietary intake and associated with energy metabolism. Both of these decisions—to largely avoid examining the fed state and to constrain metabolic interrogation to a small subset of metabolites—have severely limited the ability of studies of energy metabolism to clarify precisely how diet as a variable impacts weight regulation. Clinically, lipids are measured in the fasted condition, yet this is the period when most indices of diet and its effects on lipid metabolism are minimal. In this chapter, the principles of metabolomics are extended into two directions—input variables as food metabolite composition and output variables as the subsequent effects on post-prandial metabolism within individual humans. This approach is providing insights into the metabolic regulation associated with energy balance and obesity. The practical application of a challenge approach that measures the fluxes through specific biochemical pathways is the ability to personalize dietary recommendations based on an individual's metabolic phenotype. We propose that this approach would have a profound impact on the long-term success of diet and lifestyle-based interventions. Not only would metabolically appropriate diet and lifestyle modification be more effective in producing measurable improvements in health, perhaps even more importantly, it would increase patient acceptance and long-term adherence. Currently, people are wary of dietary recommendations because they seem to be changing every day. One day it is "beneficial" to consume eggs, the next day it is "deleterious" to consume eggs. The truth is that for some individuals eggs are beneficial while for others the cons outweigh the pros and for them egg consumption is a net negative. If we measure with accuracy and specificity the metabolic responses of individuals to specific meals and food items, and provide clear evidence that specific dietary components are causing harm whereas others are beneficial, the acceptance of recommendations will be much higher. Instead of rigidly imposed levels of acceptable intake of foods and food components that are deleterious to the health of "the average person" individuals would be free to choose foods that are palatable and enjoyable to them in doses that are metabolically appropriate for them. The success of long-term dietary and lifestyle approaches that prevent obesity and produce weight loss will ultimately depend on the acceptability of those regimens to individuals living their normal lives.

Omega-3s and Vitamin E

FREE FULLTEXT
Source; Biomed Res Int. 2014;2014:906019. doi: 10.1155/2014/906019. Epub 2014 Jul 20.
Title: The effects of vitamin E and omega-3 PUFAs on endothelial function among adolescents with

metabolic syndrome.

Authors: Ahmadi A, Gharipour M, Arabzadeh G, Moin P, Hashemipour M, Kelishadi R.

Abstract: AIM: The present study aims to explore the effects of vitamin E and omega-3 on endothelial function indicators among adolescents with metabolic syndrome.

METHOD: In a randomized, double blind, and placebo-controlled trial, 90 young individuals, aged 10 to 18 years, with metabolic syndrome were randomly assigned to receive either vitamin E tablets (400 IU/day) or omega-3 tablets (2.4 gr/day) or placebo. For assessing endothelial functional state, the serum level of vascular endothelial growth factor (VEGF) was measured by ELISA test. RESULTS: The use of omega-3 supplementation for eight weeks led to significant increase in serum HDL level compared with the group treated with vitamin E or placebo group. In this regard, no significant correlations were found between the change in VEGF and baseline levels of other markers including anthropometric indices and serum lipids. Omega-3 could significantly reduce VEGF with the presence of other baseline variables (Beta = -12.55; P = 0.012). CONCLUSION: **The administration of omega-3 can effectively improve endothelial function in adolescents with metabolic syndrome by reducing the level of serum VEGF, as a major index for atherosclerosis progression and endothelial destabilization. Omega-3 can be proposed as a VEGF antagonist for improving endothelial function in metabolic syndrome.** The clinical implications of our findings should be assessed in future studies.

Eating Slowly and Weight Loss

FREE FULLTEXT
Source: Physiol Behav. 2015 Dec 1;152(Pt B):389-
96. doi: 10.1016/j.physbeh.2015.06.038. Epub
2015 Jul 16.
Title: Effects of eating rate on satiety: A role for episodic memory?
Authors: Ferriday D, Bosworth ML, Lai S, Godinot
N, Martin N, Martin AA, Rogers PJ, Brunstrom JM.
Abstract: **Eating slowly is associated with a lower
body mass index.** However, the underlying mechanism is poorly understood. Here, our objective was
to determine whether eating a meal at a slow rate
improves episodic memory for the meal and promotes satiety. Participants (N=40) consumed a 400
ml portion of tomato soup at either a fast (1.97ml/s)
or a slow (0.50ml/s) rate. Appetite ratings were elic-
ited at baseline and at the end of the meal (satiation).
Satiety was assessed using; i) an ad libitum biscuit
'taste test' (3h after the meal) and ii) appetite ratings
(collected 2h after the meal and after the ad libitum
snack). Finally, to evaluate episodic memory for the
meal, participants self-served the volume of soup that
they believed they had consumed earlier (portion size
memory) and completed a rating of memory 'vividness'. Participants who consumed the soup slowly
reported a greater increase in fullness, both at the
end of the meal and during the inter-meal interval.
However, we found little effect of eating rate on subsequent ad libitum snack intake. Importantly, after
3h, participants who ate the soup slowly remembered
eating a larger portion. These findings show that
eating slowly promotes self-reported satiation and satiety. For the first time, they also suggest that eating
rate influences portion size memory. However, eating

slowly did not affect ratings of memory vividness and we found little evidence for a relationship between episodic memory and satiety. Therefore, we are unable to conclude that episodic memory mediates effects of eating rate on satiety.

Saturated Fat and Diabetes Prevention

Source: Circulation. 2016 Mar 22. pii: CIRCULATIONAHA.115.018410. [Epub ahead of print]
Title: Circulating Biomarkers of Dairy Fat and Risk of Incident Diabetes Mellitus Among US Men and Women in Two Large Prospective Cohorts.
Authors: Yakoob MY, Shi P, Willett WC, Rexrode KM, Campos H, Orav EJ, Hu FB, Mozaffarian D.
Abstract: BACKGROUND: -In prospective studies, relationship of self-reported consumption of dairy foods with risk of diabetes mellitus is inconsistent. Few studies have assessed dairy fat, using circulating biomarkers, and incident diabetes. We tested hypothesis that circulating fatty acid biomarkers of dairy fat, 15:0, 17:0, and t-16:1n-7, are associated with lower incident diabetes. METHODS AND RESULTS: -Among 3,333 adults aged 30-75 years and free of prevalent diabetes at baseline, total plasma and erythrocyte fatty acids were measured in blood collected in 1989-90 (Nurses' Health Study) and 1993-94 (Health Professionals Follow-Up Study). Incident diabetes through 2010 was confirmed by validated supplementary questionnaire based on symptoms, diagnostic tests, and medications. Risk was assessed using Cox proportional hazards, with

cohort findings combined by meta-analysis. During mean±SD follow-up of 15.2±5.6 years, 277 new cases of diabetes were diagnosed. In pooled multivariate analyses adjusting for demographics, metabolic risk-factors, lifestyle, diet, and other circulating fatty acids, individuals with higher plasma 15:0 had 44% lower risk of diabetes (quartiles 4 vs. 1, HR=0.56, 95%CI=0.37-0.86; P-trend=0.01); higher plasma 17:0, 43% lower risk (HR=0.57, 95%CI=0.39-0.83, P-trend=0.01); and higher t-16:1n-7, 52% lower risk (HR=0.48, 95%CI=0.33-0.70, P-trend <0.001). Findings were similar for erythrocyte 15:0, 17:0, and t-16:1n-7, although with broader CIs that only achieved statistical significance for 17:0. CONCLUSIONS: **In two prospective cohorts, higher plasma dairy fatty acid concentrations were associated with lower incident diabetes.** Results were similar for erythrocyte 17:0. Our findings highlight need to better understand potential health effects of dairy fat; and dietary and metabolic determinants of these fatty acids.

Metformin and Weight Loss

FREE FULLTEXT
Source: Drugs. 2015 Jul;75(10):1071-94. doi: 10.1007/s40265-015-0416-8.
Title: Therapeutic Use of Metformin in Prediabetes and Diabetes Prevention.
Authors: Hostalek U, Gwilt M, Hildemann S.
Abstract: People with elevated, non-diabetic, lev-

els of blood glucose are at risk of progressing to clinical type 2 diabetes and are commonly termed 'prediabetic'. The term prediabetes usually refers to high-normal fasting plasma glucose (impaired fasting glucose) and/or plasma glucose 2 h following a 75 g oral glucose tolerance test (impaired glucose tolerance). Current US guidelines consider high-normal HbA1c to also represent a prediabetic state. Individuals with prediabetic levels of dysglycaemia are already at elevated risk of damage to the microvasculature and macrovasculature, resembling the long-term complications of diabetes. Halting or reversing the progressive decline in insulin sensitivity and -cell function holds the key to achieving prevention of type 2 diabetes in at-risk subjects. Lifestyle interventions aimed at inducing weight loss, pharmacologic treatments (metformin, thiazolidinediones, acarbose, basal insulin and drugs for weight loss) and bariatric surgery have all been shown to reduce the risk of progression to type 2 diabetes in prediabetic subjects. However, lifestyle interventions are difficult for patients to maintain and the weight loss achieved tends to be regained over time. Metformin enhances the action of insulin in liver and skeletal muscle, and its efficacy for delaying or preventing the onset of diabetes has been proven in large, well-designed, randomised trials, such as the Diabetes Prevention Program and other studies. Decades of clinical use have demonstrated that metformin is generally well-tolerated and safe. We have reviewed in detail the evidence base supporting the therapeutic use of metformin for diabetes prevention.

Psychology and Weight Loss

FREE FULLTEXT
Source: Obesity (Silver Spring). 2015 Jan;23(1):7-15. doi: 10.1002/oby.20967. Epub 2014 Dec 2.
Title: NIH working group report: Innovative research to improve maintenance of weight loss.
Authors: MacLean PS, Wing RR, Davidson T, Epstein L, Goodpaster B, Hall KD, Levin BE, Perri MG, Rolls BJ, Rosenbaum M, Rothman AJ, Ryan D.

Abstract: OBJECTIVES: The National Institutes of Health, led by the National Heart, Lung, and Blood Institute, organized a working group of experts to discuss the problem of weight regain after weight loss. A number of experts in integrative physiology and behavioral psychology were convened with the goal of merging their perspectives regarding the barriers to scientific progress and the development of novel ways to improve long-term outcomes in obesity therapeutics. The specific objectives of this working group were to: (1) identify the challenges that make maintaining a reduced weight so difficult; (2) review strategies that have been used to improve success in previous studies; and (3) recommend novel solutions that could be examined in future studies of long-term weight control.
RESULTS: **Specific barriers to successful weight loss maintenance include poor adherence to behavioral regimens and physiological adaptations that promote weight regain.** A better understanding of how these behavioral and physiological barriers are related, how they vary between individuals, and how they can be overcome will lead to the development of novel strategies with improved outcomes.
CONCLUSIONS: Greater collaboration and cross-

talk between physiological and behavioral researchers is needed to advance the science and develop better strategies for weight loss maintenance.

The Rhythms of Life and Our Weight

LAN and Weight Gain

FREE FULLTEXT
Source: Am J Epidemiol. 2014 Aug 1;180(3):245-50. doi: 10.1093/aje/kwu117. Epub 2014 May 29.
Title: The relationship between obesity and exposure to light at night: cross-sectional analyses of over 100,000 women in the Breakthrough Generations Study.
Authors: McFadden E, Jones ME, Schoemaker MJ, Ashworth A, Swerdlow AJ.
Abstract: **There has been a worldwide epidemic of obesity in recent decades. In animal studies, there is convincing evidence that light exposure causes weight gain, even when calorie intake and physical activity are held constant. Disruption of sleep and circadian rhythms by exposure to light at night (LAN) might be one mechanism contributing to the rise in obesity, but it has not been well-investigated in humans.** Using multinomial logistic regression, we examined the association between exposure to LAN and obesity in questionnaire data from over 100,000 women in the Breakthrough Generations Study, a cohort study of women aged 16 years or older who were living in the United Kingdom and

recruited during 2003-2012. The odds of obesity, measured using body mass index, waist:hip ratio, waist:height ratio, and waist circumference, increased with increasing levels of LAN exposure (P < 0.001), even after adjustment for potential confounders such as sleep duration, alcohol intake, physical activity, and current smoking. We found a significant association between LAN exposure and obesity which was not explained by potential confounders we could measure. While the possibility of residual confounding cannot be excluded, the pattern is intriguing, accords with the results of animal experiments, and warrants further investigation.

Nighttime Eating and Weight Gain

FREE FULLTEXT
Source: Nutrients. 2015 Apr 9;7(4):2648-62. doi: 10.3390/nu7042648.
Title: The health impact of nighttime eating: old and new perspectives.
Authors: Kinsey AW, Ormsbee MJ.
Abstract: **Nighttime eating, particularly before bed, has received considerable attention. Limiting and/or avoiding food before night-time sleep has been proposed as both a weight loss strategy and approach to improve health and body composition.** Indeed, negative outcomes have been demonstrated in response to large mixed meals in populations that consume a majority of their daily food intake during the night. However, data is beginning to mount to suggest that negative outcomes may not

be consistent when the food choice is small, nutrient-dense, low energy foods and/or single macronutrients rather than large mixed-meals. From this perspective, it appears that a bedtime supply of nutrients can promote positive physiological changes in healthy populations. In addition, when nighttime feeding is combined with exercise training, any adverse effects appear to be eliminated in obese populations. Lastly, in Type I diabetics and those with glycogen storage disease, eating before bed is essential for survival. Nevertheless, nighttime consumption of small (~150 kcals) single nutrients or mixed-meals does not appear to be harmful and may be beneficial for muscle protein synthesis and cardiometabolic health. Future research is warranted to elucidate potential applications of nighttime feeding alone and in combination with exercise in various populations of health and disease.

Coffee and Sleep Disruption

FREE FULLTEXT
Source: Sci Transl Med. 2015 Sep 16;7(305):305ra146. doi: 10.1126/scitranslmed. aac5125.
Title: Effects of caffeine on the human circadian clock in vivo and in vitro.
Authors: Burke TM, Markwald RR, McHill AW, Chinoy ED, Snider JA, Bessman SC, Jung CM, O'Neill JS, Wright KP Jr.
Abstract: Caffeine's wakefulness-promoting and sleep-disrupting effects are well established, yet

whether caffeine affects human circadian timing is unknown. **We show that evening caffeine consumption delays the human circadian melatonin rhythm in vivo and that chronic application of caffeine lengthens the circadian period** of molecular oscillations in vitro, primarily with an adenosine receptor/cyclic adenosine monophosphate (AMP)-dependent mechanism. In a double-blind, placebo-controlled, ~49-day long, within-subject study, we found that consumption of a caffeine dose equivalent to that in a double espresso 3 hours before habitual bedtime induced a ~40-min phase delay of the circadian melatonin rhythm in humans. This magnitude of delay was nearly half of the magnitude of the phase-delaying response induced by exposure to 3 hours of evening bright light (~3000 lux, ~7 W/m(2)) that began at habitual bedtime. Furthermore, using human osteosarcoma U2OS cells expressing clock gene luciferase reporters, we found a dose-dependent lengthening of the circadian period by caffeine. By pharmacological dissection and small interfering RNA knockdown, we established that perturbation of adenosine receptor signaling, but not ryanodine receptor or phosphodiesterase activity, was sufficient to account for caffeine's effects on cellular timekeeping. We also used a cyclic AMP biosensor to show that caffeine increased cyclic AMP levels, indicating that caffeine influenced a core component of the cellular circadian clock. Together, our findings demonstrate that caffeine influences human circadian timing, showing one way that the world's most widely consumed psychoactive drug affects human physiology.

Healthy Sleep and Weight Loss

FREE FULLTEXT
Source: Diabetes. 2015 Apr;64(4):1073-80. doi: 10.2337/db14-1475.
Title: Determinants of shortened, disrupted, and mistimed sleep and associated metabolic health consequences in healthy humans.

Authors: Cedernaes J, Schiöth HB, Benedict C.

Abstract: Recent increases in the prevalence of obesity and type 2 diabetes mellitus (T2DM) in modern societies have been paralleled by reductions in the time their denizens spend asleep. Epidemiological studies have shown that disturbed sleep-comprising short, low-quality, and mistimed sleep-increases the risk of metabolic diseases, especially obesity and T2DM. Supporting a causal role of disturbed sleep, experimental animal and human studies have found that sleep loss can impair metabolic control and body weight regulation. Possible mechanisms for the observed changes comprise sleep loss-induced changes in appetite-signaling hormones (e.g., higher levels of the hunger-promoting hormone ghrelin) or hedonic brain responses, altered responses of peripheral tissues to metabolic signals, and changes in energy intake and expenditure. Even though the overall consensus is that sleep loss leads to metabolic perturbations promoting the development of obesity and T2DM, experimental evidence supporting the validity of this view has been inconsistent. This Perspective aims at discussing molecular to behavioral factors through which short, low-quality, and mistimed sleep may threaten metabolic public health. In this context, possible factors that may determine the extent to which poor sleep patterns increase the risk of metabolic pathologies within and across generations will be discussed (e.g., timing and genetics).

Melatonin and Weight Loss

Try chamomile tea before bed or low dose melatonin.

Source: Food Funct. 2014 Nov;5(11):2806-32. doi: 10.1039/c4fo00317a.
Title: Melatonin and metabolic regulation: a review.
Authors: Navarro-Alarcón M, Ruiz-Ojeda FJ, Blanca-Herrera RM, A-Serrano MM, Acuña-Castroviejo D, Fernández-Vázquez G, Agil A.

Abstract: Human life expectancy has increased over the past 50 years due to scientific and medical advances and higher food availability. However, overweight and obesity affect more than 50% of adults and 15% of infants and adolescents. There has also been a marked increase in the prevalence of metabolic syndrome in recent decades, which has been associated with a reduction in nocturnal pineal production of melatonin with aging and an increased risk of coronary diseases, type 2 diabetes mellitus (T2DM) and death. **Melatonin is currently under intensive investigation in experimental animal models of diabetes, obesity and MS at pharmacological doses (between 5 and 20 mg kg(-1) body weight), demonstrating its capacity to ameliorate the total metabolic profile and its potential as an alternative to conventional drug therapies for the disorders associated with the MS, i.e. elevated systolic blood pressure, and impairment of glucose homeostasis, plasma lipid profile, inflammation, oxidative stress, and increased body weight.** An especially significant finding is the induction by melatonin of white adipose tissue browning, which may be related to its effects against oxidative stress, uncoupling the mitochondrial bioenergetic process by enhancing the expression of uncoupled-protein-1

(UCP-1), which has been related to body weight reduction in experimental animals. Further research is required to improve knowledge of this mechanism. Clinical studies are needed with the administration of pharmacological melatonin doses, because the dose has ranged between 0.050 and 0.16 mg kg(-1) bw in most studies to date. Melatonin is a natural phytochemical, and it is also important to test its beneficial metabolic effects when consumed in functional foods.

Siesta and Healthy Weight

Source: Obes Facts. 2013;6(4):337-47. doi: 10.1159/000354746. Epub 2013 Aug 10.
Title: Association between sleeping hours and siesta and the risk of obesity: the SUN Mediterranean
Authors: Sayón-Orea C, Bes-Rastrollo M, Carlos S, Beunza JJ, Basterra-Gortari FJ, Martínez-González MA.
Abstract: OBJECTIVES:Our aim was to investigate the association between sleeping hours at night and during the siesta and the incidence of obesity in a Mediterranean cohort.
METHODS: After a median of 6.5 years of follow-up, we included 10,532 or 9,470 participants without chronic disease or obesity at baseline for analyzing the association between the incidence of obesity and nocturnal sleep duration or having siesta. Sleeping hours and siesta were assessed at baseline. Weight was recorded at baseline and every 2 years during the
160

follow-up. The outcome was the incidence of obesity during follow-up among participants with initial BMI <30 kg/m(2). RESULTS:During follow-up we observed 446 new cases of obesity in the analysis of nocturnal sleep duration. Sleeping less than 5 h at night was associated with a higher risk of becoming obese compared to sleeping between 7 and <8 h (HR 1.94; 95% CI 1.19-3.18; p for quadratic trend = 0.06) after adjusting for potential confounders. During follow-up, we observed 396 incident cases of obesity in the analysis of siesta. Those who took a siesta for 30 min/day had a 33% lower risk of becoming obese (HR 0.67; 95% CI 0.46-0.96; p for quadratic trend = 0.13) compared to those who did not take siesta. CONCLUSION:

Our results suggest that short nocturnal sleep duration could be a modifiable risk factor for obesity. It is possible that this association may be stronger among men and subjects who experienced previous weight gain. Additionally, siesta might be a novel and independent protective factor for obesity; however, confirmatory studies are needed.

The Seasons of Life and Weight Gain

FREE FULLTEXT
Source: Rockville (MD): Agency for Healthcare Research and Quality (US); 2013 Mar. Report No.: 13-EHC029-EF. AHRQ Comparative Effectiveness Reviews.
Title: Strategies to Prevent Weight Gain Among

Adults [Internet].

Authors: Hutfless S, Maruthur NM, Wilson RF, Gudzune KA, Brown R, Lau B, Fawole OA, Chaudhry ZW, Anderson CAM, Segal JB.

Excerpt: OBJECTIVES: **Adults tend to gain weight progressively through middle age. Although the average weight gain is 0.5 to 1 kg per year, this modest accumulation of weight can lead to obesity over time.** We aimed to compare the effectiveness, safety, and impact on quality of life of strategies to prevent weight gain among adults. Self-management, dietary, physical activity, orlistat and combinations of these strategies were considered.

DATA SOURCES: We searched MEDLINE®, Embase®, the Cochrane Central Register of Controlled Trials, CINAHL®, and PsycINFO® through June 2012 for published articles that were potentially eligible for this review. **REVIEW METHODS:** Two reviewers independently reviewed titles, abstracts, and articles, and included English-language articles that reported on maintenance of weight or prevention of weight gain among adults. Studies targeting a combination of weight loss with weight maintenance or weight loss exclusively were considered to be outside of the scope of this review. Trials of interventions and observational studies of approaches with at least 1 year of follow up with a weight outcome were included. Data were abstracted on measures of weight, adherence, obesity-related outcomes, safety, and quality of life. The timepoints of interest for weight outcomes were: 1 year, 2 years, 5 years, and the last reported time point after 5 years. For the other outcomes, we abstracted data only from the last reported time point on or after 1 year. We selected a meaningful difference threshold in addition to a statistically significant threshold ($p<0.05$) for the outcomes. A meaningful between group difference was defined as 0.5 kg of weight, 0.2 units of BMI (based on a 0.5-kg change for an individual with a BMI of 27), or 1 cm of waist circumference per year of follow-up. We considered an intervention or approach effective if the difference between groups met the meaningful between group difference threshold and was statistically significant. We qualitatively synthesized the studies by population, intervention, and outcome. **RESULTS:** We included 58 publications (describing 51 studies) involving 555,783 patients. Two interventions may be effective compared with no intervention at preventing weight gain with moderate strengths of evidence: workplace interventions having individual and environmental components and exercise performed at home by women with cancer. Potentially effective interventions with low strength of evidence include a clinic-based program to teach heart rate monitoring, a combination intervention for mothers of young children, small group sessions to educate college women, and physical activity among individuals at risk of cardiovascular disease and diabetes. Potentially effective approaches described in observational studies having low strength of evidence include eating meals prepared at home among college graduates and less television viewing among individuals with colorectal cancer. When reported, adherence to interventions tended to be below 80 percent. There were no adverse events among the few trials that reported on adverse events. Trial study quality tended to be poor due to knowledge of the intervention by the study personnel who measured the weight of the participants or lack of reporting on this item. This lack of blinding of the outcome assessor along with inclusion of studies that were not designed to prevent weight gain resulted in a low strength of evidence for the majority of comparisons. **CONCLUSIONS:** The literature provides some, although limited, evidence about interventions and approaches that may prevent weight gain. Although there is not strong evidence to promote a particular weight gain prevention strategy, there is no evidence that not adopting a strategy to prevent weight gain is preferable.

The Seasons of the Year and Weight Gain

Our weight gain or loss is not only is changed by our circadian, or daily, rhythms of life, but also our circumannual, or yearly, body clocks. We cannot escape the Earthly rhythms of the seasons on our basic biology.

FREE FULLTEXT
Source: Altern Med Rev. 2005 Mar;10(1):5-13.
Title: Epidemiology, etiology, and natural treatment of seasonal affective disorder.
Author: Miller AL
Abstract: **There is much more seasonal difference in higher latitudes than in lower latitudes. In a significant portion of the population of the northern United States, the shorter days of fall and winter precipitate a syndrome that can consist of depression, fatigue, hypersomnolence, hyperphagia, carbohydrate craving, weight gain, and loss of libido.** If these symptoms persist in the winter, abate as the days grow longer, and disappear in the summer, the diagnosis of seasonal affective disorder

(SAD) can be made. Many hypotheses exist regarding the biochemical mechanisms behind the predisposition toward this disease, including circadian phase shifting, abnormal pineal melatonin secretion, and abnormal serotonin synthesis. Although the mechanism(s) behind this disease is not fully known, one treatment appears to address each of the theories.Light therapy is a natural, non-invasive, effective, well-researched method of treatment for SAD. Various light temperatures and times of administration of light therapy have been studied, and a combination of morning and evening exposure appears to offer the best efficacy. Other natural methods of treatment have been studied, including L-tryptophan, Hypericum perforatum (St. John's wort), and melatonin.

FINAL THOUGHTS

Diet, the Epigenome, and Evolution

It has been shown in a Dutch population study that periods of famine had lasting effects on the epigenomics generations after the lack of nutritious food. (Veenendaal M, Painter R, de Rooij S, Bossuyt P, van der Post J, Gluckman P, Hanson M, Roseboom T. Transgenerational effects of prenatal exposure to the 1944–45 Dutch famine. BJOG2013;120:548–554.) That is, the genetic code was of these people had not changed, rather the way the environment turned on and off the expression of various genes, had been changed, and the physical effects could be seen many years later in the grandchildren.

The following articles takes this interesting thought one step further, in a large genetic study of birds and bees and biodiversity . We can extrapolate that not only does diet affect the epigenome of homo sapiens, but also our evolution as a species. From the article text: "Diet has a clear association with the diversification dynamics of birds." If the epigenome can be changed drastically in only a few years of nutritional deficit, what would a thousand years of genetic stress or lack of it do to the human genome?

FREE FULLTEXT
Source: Nature Communications, 2016; 7: 11250
DOI:10.1038/ncomms11250
Title: Omnivory in birds is a macroevolutionary sink.
Authors: Burin G, Kissling WD, Guimarães PR Jr,

Şekercioğlu ÇH, Quental TB.

Abstract: **Diet is commonly assumed to affect the evolution of species,** but few studies have directly tested its effect at macroevolutionary scales. Here we use Bayesian models of trait-dependent diversification and a comprehensive dietary database of all birds worldwide to assess speciation and extinction dynamics of avian dietary guilds (carnivores, frugivores, granivores, herbivores, insectivores, nectarivores, omnivores and piscivores). Our results suggest that omnivory is associated with higher extinction rates and lower speciation rates than other guilds, and that overall net diversification is negative. Trait-dependent models, dietary similarity and network analyses show that transitions into omnivory occur at higher rates than into any other guild. We suggest that omnivory acts as macroevolutionary sink, where its ephemeral nature is retrieved through transitions from other guilds rather than from omnivore speciation. We propose that these dynamics result from competition within and among dietary guilds, influenced by the deep-time availability and predictability of food resources.

Source: Behavioral Ecology and Sociobiology, 2016; 70 (4): 509 DOI: 10.1007/s00265-016-2067-5
Title: Honey bee foragers balance colony nutritional deficiencies.

Abstract: Honey bee colonies, foraging predominantly on a single pollen source, may encounter nutritional deficits. In the present study, we examined the nutritional resilience of honey bee colonies, testing whether foragers shift their foraging effort towards resources that complement a nutritional deficit. Eight honey bee colonies were kept in screened enclosures and fed for 1 week a pollen substitute diet deficient in a particular essential amino acid. Foragers were subsequently tested for a preference between the same diet previously fed, a different diet that was similarly deficient, or a diet that complemented the deficiency. Foragers preferred the complementary diet over the same or similar diets. Appetitive conditioning tests showed that bees were able to discriminate also between the same and similar diets. Overall, our results support the hypothesis that honey bees prefer dietary diversity, and that they do not just include novel sources but specifically target nutritionally complementary ones. Whereas we specifically focused on deficiencies in essential amino acids, we cannot rule out that bees were also complementing correlated imbalances in other nutrients, most notably essential fatty acids. The ability of honey bees to counter deficient nutrition contributes to the mechanisms which social insects use to sustain homeostasis at the colony level.

About the author:

Will is the author of twenty-five popular Kindle books in English, Spanish, and French which have gone to #1 in the USA and have sold in Canada, the United Kingdom, Spain, Mexico, Argentina, France, Germany, India, Australia, Italy, and Japan. He is a former Columbia University/NYSPI Medical Library Chief, designer, and he is a speaker of English, Spanish, French, and Portuguese.

Mr. Jiang's critically-acclaimed autobiography is "A Schizophrenic Will: A Story of Madness, A Story of Hope." Mr Jiang and his intense 20+ year struggle with schizophrenia is iconoclastic because he challenges us to think differently about stereotypes of mental illness. His peers would be world movers like Philip K. Dick, John Nash, and Elyn Saks. Most movies and media news paint one-dimensional, thinly drawn caricatures of mentally ill people, instilling fear. Refreshingly, words that could describe Mr. Jiang's life and work include: brilliant, passionate, artistic, profound, knowledgeable, inspirational, and even "wise teacher". Mr. Jiang's magnum opus in the field of psychiatry is "Guide to Natural Mental Health: Anxiety, Bipolar, Depression, Schizophrenia, and Digital Addiction: Nutrition, and Complementary Therapies" where Mr. Jiang shares deep insights into non-pharmaceutical natural strategies that are all-too-needed in this world of Big Macs and XBoxes.

William Jiang, MLS
Author Blog: http://www.mentalhealthbooks.net

Discover other titles by William Jiang, MLS

English

- A Schizophrenic Will: A Story of Madness, A Story of Hope
- Guide to Natural Mental Health: Anxiety, Bipolar, Depression, Schizophrenia, and Digital Addiction: Nutrition, and Complementary Therapies, 3rd edition
- Guide to Natural Intelligence Enhancement: The Medical Librarian's Annotated Guide
- Tackling Spanish The Easy Way
- Tackling French The Easy Way
- Tackling Portuguese the Easy Way
- My Personal Facebook Wall: 2011-2014: Sex, Lies, and My Wild and Crazy Life in New York City: A Coffee Table Book
- Facets of the Mind: Assorted Poetry and Prose of William Jiang, MLS
- How to Shop Online like A Boss: How to do Online Consumer Shopping Right in the United States
- A Historical Reader: The New York Times and Madness, 1851-1922
- The English Virtual Library
- The Medical Librarian's Guide to the Best Medicine in America

Spanish

- Entre la Esquizofrenia y Mi Voluntad: Una Historia de Locura y Esperanza - Jorge Alvarado, Traductor
- La guía del Bibliotecario Médico: Ansiedad,

Depresión, Bipolar, y Esquizofrenia: Nutrición y Terapias Complementarias, Jorge Alvarado, Traductor
- Inglés Fácilmente
- La Guía del Bibliotecario Médico: Sobre las Ciberadicciones
- La Guía del Bibliotecario Médico: la Mejor Medicina en los Estados Unidos

French

- Un Homme New Yorkais avec la Schizophrénie: Une Autobiographie